THE
CHOICE
GUIDE
TO
FOOD

DR ROSEMARY STANTON OAM is a highly respected and well-recognised expert in the fields of nutrition, dietetics and public health nutrition in Australia. She is the author of 32 books on food and nutrition, over 3500 magazine and newspaper articles, and numerous papers for scientific journals. She was awarded an Order of Australia medal for her services to community health. Rosemary lectures widely, and is a member of many government advisory committees and boards.

THE
CHOICE
GUIDE
TO
FOOD

How to look after your health,
your budget and the planet

ROSEMARY STANTON

choice BOOKS

A CHOICE book

Published by
NewSouth Publishing
University of New South Wales Press Ltd
University of New South Wales
Sydney NSW 2052
AUSTRALIA
newsouthpublishing.com

© Rosemary Stanton 2011
First published 2011

10 9 8 7 6 5 4 3 2 1

National Library of Australia
Cataloguing-in-Publication entry
    Title: The CHOICE guide to food: How to look after your
        health, your budget and the planet/Rosemary Stanton.
    ISBN: 9 781 74223 294 2 (pbk.)
    Notes: Includes index.
    Subjects: Food.
        Diet.
        Health.
    Dewey Number: 641.3

Design Di Quick
Images iStockphoto, Dreamstime
Cover design Design by Committee
Printer Ligare

This book is printed on paper using fibre supplied from
plantation or sustainably managed forests.

Contents

For Peter, with thanks

MY FOOD PHILOSOPHY IS SIMPLE: fresh, healthy and delicious meals. I want to know where my food comes from and that its production shows respect for the earth's limited resources. Foods need to be 'real' rather than manufactured 'lookalikes'. As our knowledge grows, I am delighted to discover that choosing foods with environmental sustainability in mind dovetails beautifully with a healthful diet. Over many years working as a public health nutritionist and sitting on numbers of government committees and advisory boards, I am also conscious of the importance of scientific evidence and of the battle to get sound ideas across when we're constantly bombarded with an endless stream of theories about foods and dietary patterns being 'good' or 'bad'.

Eggs are damned for their cholesterol but then get a Heart Foundation tick of approval. Butter is banished from the table by many, and others maintain margarine is worse. Sugar is called 'sweet poison' and some claim it is more harmful to health than fat. Television devotes whole programs to the antioxidants in goji berries, cranberries or some other super fruit. Chocolate has become a health food – but is it really? Products such as quinoa, ginseng and royal jelly are hailed as heroes that can deliver us from health problems. Others want us to stop eating rice and potatoes because of their high glycaemic index. Red wine is 'good' because it helps the heart (and maybe the brain) but 'bad' because it increases the risk of some cancers, including breast cancer. We're told of the health properties of oils but warned we must not use them for frying. High-protein diets with loads of red meat are promoted even as the World Cancer Research Fund publishes findings that red meat increases the risk of bowel cancer. Soy is good one day, dreadful the next. Some say organic foods are a must; others claim they are not worth the extra cost.

And so it goes on – countless confusing claims. Shopping is now a nightmare for the health conscious wending their way through the 30 000 items in the modern supermarket, trying to read the fine print on labels and remember which items are now in the good books.

Of course, outrageous claims are not new, but the old snake oil tales have expanded with the range of products available. And as new media reach into our lives, the hype has reached new heights. Google almost any topic and you're confronted with thousands of entries, espousing theories that may be correct or have little basis in fact. How are we supposed to know who to believe? Even medical experts differ on matters related to food, nutrition and health – and you can find a study somewhere to support almost any theory.

I blame vested interests for much of the confusion. The internet is a dream for sellers and spreaders of 'good' and 'bad' information. Much research is sponsored by companies that stand to gain from proving particular theories – theories that are then spread through PR releases whose content may bear little relationship to the actual research results.

The science of nutrition doesn't make it easy either, mainly because many other factors can interact with the effects of food. What we eat and drink may sometimes be less relevant than the genes we inherited. It's also worth remembering that, apart from breast milk in the first six months of life, no single food can meet all our body's needs and no one food is essential. Some foods are so good for health that they deserve a place in each day's diet. Others can be hazardous, although it is always 'the dose that makes the poison'.

So how do we make rational choices about our diets? My aim here has been to take a critical overview of the evidence about many of the foods, drinks and supplements that line our supermarket shelves. In weighing up the strengths and weaknesses of different theories, I have tried to provide balanced, sensible, commonsense advice so that shopping and eating are simpler, healthier, more enjoyable – and above all, more sustainable.

The basics

of healthy eating

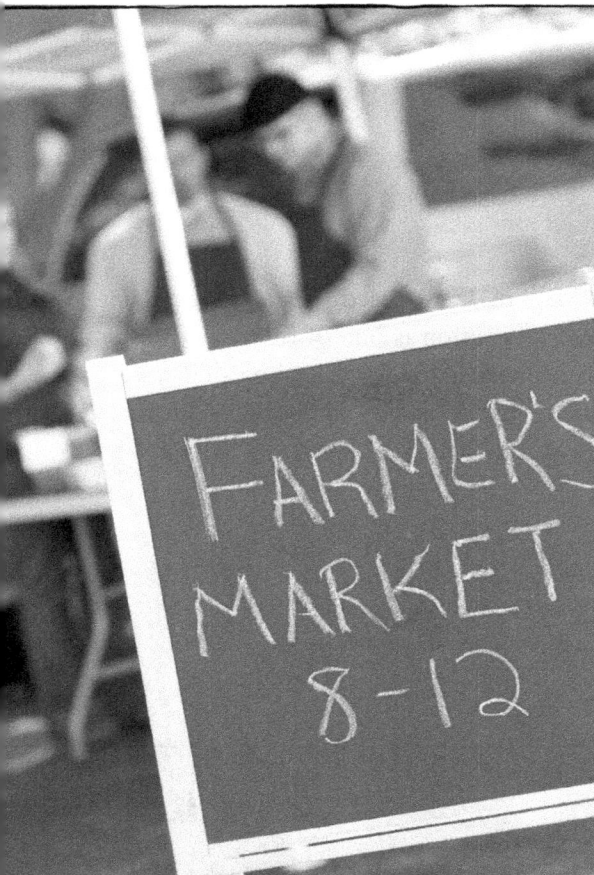

NUTRITIONISTS ARE SOMETIMES accused of changing their minds – indeed, countering that perception is one of the reasons for writing this book – but the basic ingredients for a healthy diet have hardly changed in over 50 years. The easiest way to choose foods for good health is to select from each of the five food groups:

- vegetables, including legumes
- fruit
- cereal grains and wholegrain products made from them
- fish or lean meat or poultry or eggs, nuts, seeds and legumes
- milk, cheese and yoghurt or calcium-enriched substitutes.

Fruit and vegetables were once combined as a single food group, but current research shows they are different enough to warrant separate groups. The old 'fats' group has been dropped, although not forgotten. Seeds, legumes, grains and nuts and fish are all sources of essential fatty acids, and are now recognised as just that – essential.

Healthy eating involves eating more of some foods and less of others. The foods we need provide us with nutrients such as protein, essential fatty acids, vitamins, minerals and dietary fibre. Plant-based foods also contain a huge range of components called phytonutrients (Greek *phyto* means 'plant') that contribute to health and longevity. Contrary to popular belief, these plant components are not simply 'antioxidants' – they have a much wider range of action.

Almost everyone can also deal with small quantities of salt and refined sugars and less desirable forms of fat. Large amounts can contribute to various health problems.

The exact quantities of essential foods and 'extras' we consume depend on age, our amount of lean muscle tissue, physical activity and growth (relevant in childhood and adolescence, and during pregnancy). As we get older, our need for kilojoules usually decreases, although there may be an increased need for some minerals, vitamins, dietary fibre and essential fats. This leaves less room for junk foods. A similar situation occurs in pregnancy where more essential nutrients are needed, without much appreciable increase in kilojoules.

Take a look in the mirror. Everything you see was once in your food. Our genes and many environmental factors play a role in the way we look and what size and shape we are, but food provides the fuel to keep us going and the material to repair the tiny bits of damage that occur just through normal living. Choosing healthy foods in the right quantity for our size, stage of life and physical activity is vital to keeping the body in good running order. And although the amazing resilience of the human body allows for occasional lapses, a constant diet of junk foods almost always takes its toll on health.

So how do we choose a healthy diet? Throughout most of human history, people have simply eaten what they could kill or forage. Some dietary zealots maintain we should revert to the way our Palaeolithic ancestors ate, although they rarely suggest we return to living in caves and wearing animal skins for clothes. Around 10 000 years ago, the establishment of agriculture led to major changes in the foods we consume, but diet-related health problems have increased only in the last 50 or so years. Over this more recent period, major changes have involved adopting a sedentary way of life and dramatically increasing our food choices. In the 1960s, most Australians could choose from 600 to 800 foods, many available only seasonally. We shopped in small stores, visiting the butcher, grocer and fruit and vegetable shop, usually taking a shopping list and asking the shopkeeper for what we needed. By the late 1960s, affluence and technology combined to change our food supply. Supermarkets sprang up to showcase the new products developed by food technologists and as we were able to walk around and take foods from shelves we were offered more and more. Processed foods increased in number, but so did fresh produce with new vegetables and different cuts of meat and chicken introduced to fit the new recipes being promoted in magazines and newspapers. These days, modern supermarkets stock about 30 000 items of food and drink. The increased range includes some healthy foods and new versions of some fresh fruits and vegetables, but the overwhelming expansion has been in ready-to-eat processed junk foods and drinks. A typical Australian supermarket now offers about 1800 different snack foods, many of which are also available wherever we work, relax or even buy fuel for our cars.

This combination of a sedentary lifestyle and the ready availability of junk foods and drinks has resulted in over 60 per cent of the adult population now classified as overweight or obese. Since the mid-1980s, the incidence of overweight has doubled. Obesity rates have tripled. A quarter of Australian children are now overweight or obese.

As the population has grown fatter, so has the incidence of type 2 diabetes increased dramatically, with experts estimating that one Australian in 12 now has the disease, once called 'adult-onset' diabetes. The name was changed to type 2 diabetes when the disorder appeared for the first time in young people. Rates of type 2 diabetes are continuing to increase so rapidly that this chronic disease threatens to overwhelm future health budgets with its complications – which include heart attack and stroke, and problems with kidneys, eyes, and peripheral circulation. Many other health problems are also related to excess body fat, including cardiovascular disease, some common types of cancer and dementia.

There is no mystery as to why we are growing fatter: we are eating more and moving less. Physical activity burns up kilojoules and is also important because it helps regulate the appetite. The benefits of activity are easy to see with animals. Most animals that roam freely and eat at will don't get fat. To fatten them up, farmers put them into small areas, pens or cages. This reduces their activity levels, their appetite control mechanism fails, and they eat more. This is similar to humans adopting a sedentary way of life, with easy-to-eat kilojoules, sugar-laden drinks and alcohol combining to further disrupt our normal appetite control.

We actually eat much the same weight of food as previous generations, but modern processed meals and snacks are more energy dense, due to their greater concentration of sugars, fats and refined starches. One reason why dietary guidelines recommend we eat more fresh fruits and vegetables is that their natural fibre and high water content add bulkiness without kilojoules.

Reading a food label

If you read every food label before buying anything, shopping would take a long time. However, many people do read the labels on new or unfamiliar products, and they contain some useful facts. In Australia, every food label must provide some basic information, including:

- the name of the product
- the name and address of the manufacturer, packer, importer or vendor
- the country of origin
- identification of where the food was produced and a 'lot' or 'batch' number so the food can be traced to its packaging plant
- a 'use by' or 'best before' date, or the date of packaging if the food has a long shelf life
- a nutrition information panel
- a list of ingredients, in descending order of their weight in the product
- the percentage of any ingredient mentioned in the the name of the product or considered a characterising ingredient (such as cocoa solids in chocolate).

'USE BY' DATE

All packaged foods that have a shelf life of two years or less, and are sold in shops or for catering purposes in restaurants, canteens or self-catering institutions, must carry a 'best before' statement, unless the food needs to be eaten within a certain period for health or safety reasons, in which case it must carry a 'use by' date.

Foods that have a 'use by' date may not be sold after this date as consumption could carry a health or safety risk. Foods with a 'best before' date can be sold after the date has passed, as long as they are still fit for human consumption.

THE NUTRITION INFORMATION PANEL (NIP)

This is the place to check how much energy, protein, fat, saturated fat, total carbohydrate, sugars and sodium a product contains. And if a manufacturer makes a claim about any other nutrient – for example, vitamins, minerals or dietary fibre – that nutrient must also be added to the NIP. There are also laws about which foods can have added vitamins and minerals – which prevent companies adding vitamins to jelly beans, for example. Some manufacturers get around this by marketing sweets with added vitamins and minerals as 'therapeutic goods' rather than foods.

Products that make a claim about the nature of the fats they contain (for example, polyunsaturated, monounsaturated or trans fats) must also list the percentage quantities of those fats.

When checking the NIP, compare products using the per 100 g or 100 mL columns rather than the serving size columns. Serving sizes can be deceptive, as manufacturers can pick whatever quantity they like. This may be very different from what most people would consume. For example, most people would eat more muesli than is contained in the 30 g serving often listed on the NIP label. The serving size of some products also fails the test of common sense. If a dairy dessert comes in a 200 mL container, it is absurd to list the serving size as 150 mL. Is anyone really likely to leave the last little bit? Some margarines list a 5 g serving size, except for those with added plant sterols, where claims of a 'reduction in cholesterol absorption' are only valid with higher quantities. Serving sizes are clearly manipulated by manufacturers and need to be taken with a grain of (the proverbial) salt.

INGREDIENT LIST

The ingredient list is probably the most valuable piece of information on a food label. All ingredients must be listed and the order of prominence gives some idea of what you are buying. If sugar is near the top of the ingredient list, the product is probably not worth buying, whereas sugar listed among minor ingredient along with yeast or a flavouring is of little concern. Take care if the ingredient list has several sugars (such as raw sugar, honey, glucose, molasses, maltose, or anything else ending in 'ose') as this usually means the total sugar content is high.

Genetically modified (GM) ingredients containing protein must be listed, but GM sugars and fats escape this scrutiny. The label must declare if any ingredient or food has been subjected to irradiation.

PERCENTAGE LABELLING

The percentage of any ingredient included in a product's name (for example chicken soup, wholemeal bread, peanut butter) must be included on the food label. This helps shoppers know what they are buying and assists with assessing true value. For example, if two brands of peanut butter sell for the same price, but one is 100 per cent peanuts whereas the other has only 85 per cent peanuts (with the remaining 15 per cent consisting of added sugar, salt and several emulsifiers or other additives), it's easy to know which is the better buy. Dried cranberries are another example where the percentage of the main ingredient is relevant to value. If you want cranberries rather than sugar, paying $4.50 for a packet of dried cranberries with 60 per cent fruit is a better buy than the same size packet costing $4, but with only 50 per cent fruit. Or check out jars of crushed garlic. One with 50 per cent garlic is a poor buy because you know you are paying for half a jar of water, sugar and food acid. For a far better buy, go to the vegetable section where you get fresh bulbs of garlic with no additives. Soup labels are particularly informative, particularly when you discover that some brands of chicken soup now have less than 1 per cent chicken.

Arithmetic skills are handy for percentage labelling but vigilance may also be needed for some spreads, confectionery bars and ice confections claiming a high percentage of fruit. The 'fruit' may be in the form of concentrated pear or apple juice with little more than the sugar retained from the original fruit. Such 'fruit' has virtually none of the original nutritional assets of the whole fruit.

Australian authorities impose some percentage standards on foods judged to be 'iconic'. A meat pie must contain 25 per cent meat (offal can be added but must be identified); sausages must have 50 per cent meat flesh; jam must contain at least 40 per cent of the fruit mentioned on the label (if not, it must be called a 'spread'); while ice cream must have 10 per cent milk fat or give up the name 'ice cream' in favour of 'ice confection'.

'FREE' CLAIMS

Many food labels proclaim a product is 'x% something free', usually applied to fat, as in '93% fat free'. A Code of Practice exists to provide guidelines for using such marketing terms, but the code is regularly flouted and because it is not mandatory there is no penalty for deception. The voluntary code states that '%fat-free' should only be used on foods that fit the mandatory requirement to be called 'low fat' (less than 3 g fat/100 g or less than 1.5g fat/100 mL for liquid products). It's not difficult to fill a shopping basket with products that ignore the code. With published evidence of widespread flouting of the code now available, a recent labelling review commissioned by the federal government has recommended stricter legislated rules.

'Cholesterol free' claims can also be misleading. Cholesterol is part of the structure of animal tissue. It does not occur in plants, so 'cholesterol free' claims for foods such as avocadoes or rolled oats or vegetable oil spreads are absurd. In any case, most excess blood cholesterol does not come from consuming cholesterol in foods, but is produced within the body when the diet is high in saturated fat.

Some teas claim to be '97% caffeine free'. This is also nonsense, since regular tea has only 3 per cent caffeine. The implication that these teas are different or have had most of their caffeine removed is misleading.

PERCENTAGE DAILY INTAKE

It pays to be wary of front-of-pack 'thumbnails' describing the percentage daily intake (%DI) for energy, protein, fats, sugars, sodium and a range of minerals and vitamins. This scheme has no official government

16

backing and independent researchers have shown that the %DI scheme can be confusing, and could even be misleading for many people.

The %DI does not include the letter 'R', which would reflect the official recommended dietary intakes (RDI). RDIs are set by a panel of experts and are assigned only where sufficient high quality evidence exists. RDIs are also specific for different groups within the community. By contrast, %DI uses a variety of figures and ignores the fact that a single value for energy or any nutrient will not apply to the whole population. Manufacturers also decide on the serving size they will use for %DI, and this sometimes varies for products with essentially the same use, such as margarine spreads. This may be different from what most people would consume and is not even consistently applied to similar products. The value currently used for %DI for energy is appropriate for a non-overweight male (a minority group). The protein %DI represents the needs for an average adult. The %DIs for various fats are hard to fathom, especially as there are no standard RDIs for these; appropriate RDI values depend on many factors, including size, age and activity level. Nor do we have a recommendation for sugar intake, although authorities such as the World Health Organization recommend that added sugar should contribute less than 10 per cent of daily kilojoules – a level considerably lower than the industry uses for its %DI. The sodium figure used for %DI is the upper limit recommended by health authorities, not the much lower desirable intake.

The federal government's recent labelling review noted that %DI is confusing, uses inconsistent serving sizes, is based on adult requirements, and the use of percentages is confusing for the majority of people. Even those with higher level skills will find it challenging to recall the percentage of each nutrient in what they have already consumed that day. In any case, with some nutrients such as sodium, the goal is to consume only a small quantity. There is no evidence that the %DI scheme encourages people to choose a healthier diet.

Fats

Chemists classify fats by their chemical structure as saturated or unsaturated fats. For years, nutritionists were concerned about a high-fat diet contributing to high levels of fats in the blood and resulting in clogged arteries. That concern led to recommendations to avoid high-fat foods. Nutritionists were recommending leaner meats, reduced-fat milk and fewer pastries, cakes, biscuits and fried foods. The processed food industry, however, took the low-fat mantra to mean that foods could contain anything as long as the fat level was reduced. This led to thousands of new foods being produced with fat replaced by sugar or a range of starches technically engineered to produce a similar mouth-feel to fat. Unfortunately, many of these foods had at least as many kilojoules as the foods they were meant to replace. The public took to the low-fat foods with great enthusiasm and it was common for people to think it was fine to eat junk foods such as jelly beans, marshmallows or many desserts as long as they carried a low-fat or reduced-fat tag.

A backlash also occurred, especially as the population continued to grow fatter as low-fat products proliferated. Many people began to claim that carbohydrates were the real problem whereas fats were 'essential'. Let's sort out the facts.

ESSENTIAL FATTY ACIDS

Some fats found in foods such as fish and other seafood, nuts and seeds, legumes, oats and liquid vegetable oils contain essential fatty acids, which *are* essential. We all need to include them in our diet. However, it is misleading to translate this into statements such as 'we must have some fat', or 'fat is good'. The essential fatty acids are not found in many commonly consumed high-fat foods, which generally contain less desirable saturated fats.

SATURATED FATS

There is some dispute about the healthfulness of saturated fats, mainly because some can be more undesirable than others. Infants certainly need these fats because their rapid growth demands a concentrated source of kilojoules. In general, however, saturated fats are not essential to health. Many research studies find that most people would be better off with less saturated fat than is commonly consumed, and possibly more of the essential fatty acids. Fatty meats, dairy fats and the solid frying fats used in many commercially-produced fried foods, pastries,

18

crisps and other snacks, breakfast bars and confectionery do not meet our needs for essential fatty acids.

UNSATURATED FATS

Unsaturated fats can be described as either monounsaturated or poly-unsaturated. These fats have the same kilojoule count as saturated fats but they do not raise blood cholesterol and are generally considered to be 'good' fats. Most foods contain a mixture of different fats, but are generally known by their predominant type. Monounsaturated fats are the predominant fats in olive oil, most nuts, canola and oats. Poly-unsaturated fats can be divided into two main classes: omega 3s and omega 6s, with the distinction being based on their chemical structure. Essential fatty acids are polyunsaturated and include:

- an omega 6 fatty acid called linoleic acid (found in seeds such as sunflower or sesame, walnuts and many vegetable oils)
- an omega 3 fatty acid called alpha linolenic acid (found in foods such as linseeds, walnuts, oats and soybeans)
- a long chain omega 3 fatty acid found in fish and other seafood, with smaller quantities in meat from grass-fed sheep and cattle and some eggs.

The omega 3 and omega 6 fats need to be in balance. For most western diets, this means less omega 6 fats and more omega 3s.

TRANS FATS

Some unsaturated fats are also known as trans fats. Several of them are found naturally in meat and dairy products and are generally considered harmless. However one trans fat that doesn't occur in nature is of concern, an industrially produced substance that has no redeeming health features. This nasty trans fat is called elaidic acid and it's produced when vegetable oils are subjected to a process known as partial hydrogenation. When you hear complaints from medical scientists about trans fat, this is the one that worries them. Partial hydrogenation turns a liquid oil into a solid fat (elaidic acid) that has a longer shelf life and produces a crisp texture in baked, fried and crunchy foods. This fat also gives foods like muffins, cakes and pastries a desirable texture in the mouth. To add to its technological appeal, trans fat also produces a spreadable consistency in margarine spreads made from vegetable oils.

Somewhat ironically, this trans fat increased in the food supply when food labelling laws required processed foods to label their saturated fat content. Before compulsory labelling, many foods contained saturated fat derived from animal fats, palm and palm kernel oils or hydrogenated vegetable oils. Once labelling was required, many companies switched to a partial hydrogenation process since the resulting trans fat was technically 'unsaturated' and so did not fall under the labelling requirement.

In terms of its effects on the body, research shows clearly that elaidic acid increases LDL ('bad') blood cholesterol (as does saturated fat), decreases HDL ('good') cholesterol (unlike saturated fat) and also increases triglycerides and several other undesirable forms of fat. Elaidic acid also promotes inflammatory reactions in the body. Since it has no redeeming nutritional features, health authorities around the world have agreed there is no safe level of consumption.

Denmark, Austria and New York State have effectively legislated to eliminate industrially-produced trans fat, and labelling is mandatory in some other countries. Research in Denmark has shown that fears labelling will encourage companies to revert to using saturated fats are unfounded.

After intense lobbying from nutritionists, Australian margarine manufacturers removed trans fats from their products more than 10 years ago. However, some commercially-produced fried foods – doughnuts, muffins, chicken nuggets, snack foods, some crumbed foods, crackers, pastries and confectionery – still contain trans fat. The recent labelling review recommends full labelling but Food Standards Australia New Zealand (FSANZ), the official food authority, does not consider that 'average' trans fat consumption is high enough to warrant the change.

Processed foods

Apart from fresh fruit and vegetables, most foods are subjected to some form of processing. For meat, poultry and fish, processing involves butchering the animals and presenting trimmed cuts of flesh. Milk is now pasteurised (a technique that has dramatically reduced milk-borne infections); a great deal of milk is made into yoghurts and cheeses.

Grains are ground into flour. When flour is combined with water, yeast and a little salt, the resulting bread is a processed food. Many foods, raw or cooked, are frozen or canned in water, brine or syrup. Some people argue that packaging (bagging or wrapping in plastic) is also a form of processing that generally extends the safe life of the food. These are all simple processes that have been used for many years.

Some more modern processing methods are more involved. For example, processing 'deli' meats may involve the mechanical removal of meat or chicken from bones, with the resulting slurry solidified in a 'bath' of brine and mineral salts.

STARCHES

Food technologists have developed a range of refined starches that they claim provide adhesion, binding, clouding, dusting, stabilisation of emulsions, encapsulation, better flow, strengthen foams, assist gelling, glazing and moisture retention, allow moulding and shaping, prevent foods going stale, and stabilise and thicken them.

Among the uses of these refined starches are: providing a smooth or creamy texture in the mouth to desserts, yoghurt and instant puddings; keeping particles suspended in salad dressings and drinks; preventing cakes from crumbling; retaining water in products such as sausages, chicken breast and some deli meats; thickening and giving a smooth shiny appearance to marinades and mayonnaise; producing transient gels in frozen low-fat ice creams so they feel like cream melting in your mouth; providing crispness or stickiness in cereals, pastries and con-fectionery or holding sesame seeds on crackers; providing soft or hard textures to lollies.

None of these starches has any positive nutritional value. Most provide kilojoules and although they increase the range of processed foods available, they do so by diluting the quantity of real ingredients.

ADDITIVES

Many people are concerned about the use of food additives. People who suffer from food intolerances may react adversely to additives such as flavour enhancers, particular preservatives or particular colourings. From my perspective, the potential problems are less likely to be due

THE BASICS OF HEALTHY EATING

to the additives themselves than to the kinds of foods and eating patterns they make possible. True, some additives help make foods safer, but many others merely facilitate the invention of more junk foods and drinks. Avoiding foods with additives will often improve the diet because the foods that contain additives are also responsible for most of our intake of trans and saturated fats, sugar, refined starches and salt. The bulk of these problem components of foods are consumed because additives make them attractive.

Countries have worked together in the Codex Alimentarius Commission (established by the World Health Organization) to assign numbers to the several thousand food additives. Each country decides what they will permit to be added to their foods, but additive numbers are constant across the world. Number 621, for example, is monosodium glutamate (MSG) everywhere from Norway to New Zealand; the artificial sweetener aspartame is always 951. The number of any additive may be omitted if the full name is used. Some colourings or preservatives or other additives permitted in one country may be banned in others.

In Australia, additives must first be approved by FSANZ, which publishes a list of permitted additives by name and number, available on the FSANZ website or as a small booklet. Scientists at FSANZ also decide on an acceptable daily intake (ADI) for all additives and, on the basis of likely consumption, then decide which foods can carry particular additives. They also carry out occasional surveys to estimate the current likely intake of some additives to check that high users do not approach the ADI. When surveys of artificial sweeteners, for example, revealed that some people were approaching the ADI for cyclamates, FSANZ lowered the permitted level of cyclamates for use in cordials and other beverages.

Food additives are classified as:

- acid regulators (help reduce growth of bacteria)
- anti-caking agents (prevent salt and other powders from clumping together)
- antioxidants (added to fats to prevent rancidity)
- bulking agents (often used with artificial sweeteners which lack the usual bulk of sugar)
- colourings (may be natural or artificial)

- emulsifiers (stop oil separating out)
- firming agents (keep substances dispersed evenly in solid and semi-solid foods)
- flavour enhancers (increase the flavour and thereby mask the lack of 'real' ingredients)
- flavourings (may be natural or artificial)
- foaming agents (keep gases evenly distributed in soft drinks)
- gelling agents (change the texture of foods by forming gels)
- glazing agents (such as waxes used on apples)
- humectants (used to stop foods like icing on cakes from drying out)
- preservatives (designed to stop foods going bad)
- raising agents (used in cakes and other baked goods)
- sweeteners (used in place of sugar)
- thickeners (various starches).

A full list of food additives permitted in Australia is available from FSANZ – see <foodstandards.gov.au>. The list includes only those additives approved for use in this country. Gaps in the list represent additives that are not used in Australia, either because permission has been refused or simply because no food company has yet applied to use a particular additive.

Choosing an environmentally friendly diet

Eating according to the dietary guidelines could reduce our carbon footprint as well as improving health. The guidelines recommend cutting the consumption of highly processed foods and drinks and reducing meat consumption. Some packaging improves shelf life and can reduce food waste, but much of it wraps around fast foods, drinks and snacks that create havoc for health and the environment. Almost two thirds of all packaging in Australia is for food products.

A diet that is good for the health of the body is remarkably similar to what we should choose for the health of the planet. Instead of continually emphasising the need to lose weight or eat less fat or sugar, we could take a positive approach and concentrate on eating in ways that are consistent with the principles of environmental sustainability. Changing our food choices to reduce our carbon footprint may be a better motivator for healthier food choices than emphasising kilojoules.

Each of us can reduce our carbon footprint by consuming and wasting less, and choosing more locally grown fresh foods. Each part of the food industry aims to sell more, but adopting a new mindset of frugality – using tap water and buying minimally packaged and processed foods, and reducing our purchases of junk foods and drinks because they are a waste of resources (including money) – is one way we can help preserve the local and global environment and at the same time decrease obesity and other health problems related to our excess consumption.

Changing the *kinds* of foods we consume is important. Moving meat away from the centre of the plate and choosing more plant-based foods supplemented with a smaller quantity of meat from sustainable sources will also help in reducing our carbon footprint. Almost 18 per cent of greenhouse gas emission in Australia is related to beef production. Over 800 000 hectares of Australia's agricultural land is used to produce the 1.5 million tonnes of grain and 815 000 tonnes of roughage that beef cattle consume. In the United States, half of all grain and legumes grown is fed to animals. Worldwide, more than a third of crops go to animals. If grains and legumes were solely grown for and distributed to humans, we could wipe out starvation.

Clearing land for cattle and sheep also creates environmental problems. Switching to more modest portions of meat produced by cattle and sheep that graze on otherwise unproductive land would help reduce greenhouse gas emissions from livestock.

The major problem caused by cattle and sheep involves their production of methane – a greenhouse gas with over 20 times the warming effects of carbon dioxide. Researchers are trying to breed animals with different gut microbes and feeding regimes that will reduce methane emissions in the animals' burps, but success so far has been modest, with reductions of only about 6 per cent in emissions from cattle. Pigs, poultry and kangaroos do not produce methane. Pigs and chickens require less land than sheep and cattle and are also more efficient converters of food to flesh. Kangaroos do not require land to be cleared and their long feet cause far less erosion and mineral losses from soil than the hard cloven hoofs of sheep and cattle. Kangaroo meat is also a good source of essential fatty acids and protein and has high levels of iron, zinc and vitamin B12.

The bonuses in choosing an environmentally friendly pattern of eating include benefits to the household budget as we cut down on waste and choose foods lower in the food chain (more plant-based foods with less processing and packaging). This way of eating also brings possibilities of greater enjoyment as we savour the flavour of fresh local foods in season, and we have the bonus of health advantages from smaller quantities of red meats and fewer packaged foods with their added sugar, starches and fats.

A tax applied according to the carbon footprint of foods would be one way to improve the diet. Such a tax might also be less unpopular than the junk food tax that has been proposed by almost every inquiry into ways to change consumption patterns. People might see a reduction in their purchases of highly processed and packaged foods for the sake of the planet and the future of their children and grandchildren as a positive step.

The most environmentally friendly foods just happen to be the healthiest choices. Promoting this type of diet is now on the agenda in Sweden, Germany, Switzerland, the United Kingdom and Australia. A report from the UK's Sustainable Consumption Commission concluded that reducing meat and dairy foods, eating fewer fatty and sugary foods and wasting less food would make major changes towards creating a more sustainable diet.

Wasted food also costs dearly. Current figures estimate that one third of the food produced in the world is wasted, by pests and climatic conditions in developing countries and by over-purchasing and throwing out food in developed countries. The Australia Institute calculated that Australians throw away $5.3 billion worth of food annually (2004 data). More recent calculations show that the 7.5 million tonnes of food discarded each year in Australia would be enough to give three hearty meals to 13.6 million people every day for a year. These are horrific figures when you consider that the Australian population totals only 22.5 million. As well as the waste itself, food added to landfill generates methane gas – every kilogram of food left to decompose produces the equivalent of 1 kilogram of greenhouse gases.

On the topic of landfill, even with current recycling efforts, 65 per cent of the plastic water bottles purchased in Australia are not recycled.

Worldwide, over 400 billion plastic bottles are added to landfill each year. It's particularly silly that most bottled water is sold in countries with a safe water supply, while millions of people in less developed countries die each year because they have only contaminated water to drink. Bottled water may be a healthier drink than sweetened drinks, but it is environmentally unacceptable and absurdly expensive, with some 'designer waters' selling for up to 10000 times the cost of tap water.

FOOD MILES AND OTHER ISSUES

The concept of 'food miles' represents the distance food travels from paddock to plate. The term was introduced in the early 1990s by Professor Tim Lang as part of his strategy to encourage people to think about where their food came from. Did it make sense for foods produced in the UK, for example, to travel to other European countries while the same countries shipped similar products back to the UK? In Australia, trucks carrying chickens from Queensland to Victoria can literally pass trucks carrying chickens from Victoria to Queensland. Fruit and vegetables produced in Orange in New South Wales used to be sent to the markets in Sydney and then back to supermarkets in Orange. A Victorian study in 2008 estimated the food miles and carbon emissions for a food basket containing 29 commonly purchased foods – the total distance travelled was 70803 kilometres.

Such crazy systems led to considerations of 'food miles' and subsequent moves to sell local produce close to where it is grown. Locavore groups, begun in the United States in 2005, aimed at serving only food grown within a 100 mile (160 kilometre) radius. It's a worthy aim that stresses the need to think about where food comes from, although it may be more applicable in some places than others.

The environmental arguments need to consider a broad range of issues. Some foods can be produced with a lower carbon footprint in particular areas, for example where soils are fertile and require less fertiliser and where adequate rainfall means less need to deplete scarce water resources through the use of irrigation. Bulk transport for some products can also lower the carbon footprint. This is currently occurring in the UK with some supermarkets importing bulk containers of wine from Australia and bottling the wine on arrival. Without the need to transport heavy glass bottles across the world, the carbon emissions for these wines are reduced by 80 per cent. Lamb produced in New Zealand where the animals graze on grass has also been shown to have a much smaller footprint, even when frozen and exported to Britain, than intensively reared, grain-fed lamb produced closer to the UK market.

Supplements

There are times when the dietary intake of some nutrients may be inadequate and supplements may be required. This is especially relevant for the frail aged whose reduced ability to absorb some nutrients can be compensated for with larger quantities of nutrients taken as supplements. Anyone who cannot eat regular foods or whose diet is severely restricted because of food allergies or intolerances will also benefit from appropriate supplements.

During pregnancy, supplements may be prescribed as a safeguard to ensure the higher needs are provided. Iron supplements were once routinely prescribed during pregnancy, and will be vital if a woman's iron levels are low at the beginning of her pregnancy. However, research now shows that the absorption of iron in foods can increase during pregnancy and iron should only be taken where it is genuinely needed. Iodine supplements are important during pregnancy in many parts of Australia where the soils are low in iodine and levels in foods are consequently inadequate to meet the increased demands of pregnancy.

For the majority of the population, however, if the diet is so poor that supplements are needed, the obvious choice is to make better choices from the range of nutritious foods available.

Vitamin D may be an exception. We normally make vitamin D from the action of sunlight on skin. This requires only about 10–15 minutes exposure of the head, neck and arms. However, for women whose culture or religion forbids them exposing their skin, and also frail aged people who cannot go outside, there is virtually no way to get enough vitamin D without taking a supplement. The breast-fed babies of veiled women also need a supplement of this vitamin as do those who cannot risk exposure to the sun because of a high risk of skin cancer.

The most commonly consumed supplement is vitamin C, taken to prevent or reduce the symptoms of the common cold. Yet more than 30 studies comparing vitamin C with a placebo have shown the supplement is rarely effective. The only studies showing any effect involved soldiers under extreme physical duress in sub-Arctic conditions or elite skiers training at altitude.

Calcium tablets are also popular, but several recent studies show they may increase risk of kidney problems and heart disease. Foods high in calcium do not pose similar risks because their calcium is more slowly absorbed. More studies are needed to resolve possible problems with calcium supplements, but the safest option is to choose foods to provide calcium.

Some people take multi-vitamins as a form of nutritional insurance. This is usually a waste of money, but is unlikely to be harmful. However, supplements are a poor substitute for nutritious foods and lack the complex and valuable components found in foods. Some nutrients also need to work together and isolating a single nutrient and taking it as a supplement can have unfortunate consequences. When several studies found that smokers who ate more fruit and vegetables were less likely to get lung cancer, trials were set up giving smokers either the vitamins found in fruits and vegetables or placebo pills. In one large study of 29 000 smokers, those given supplements of beta carotene (a carotenoid compound that the body converts to vitamin A) developed more lung cancer than those taking either extra fruit and vegetables or a placebo. Other studies that were occurring broke their coded results and found a similar problem.

Many other studies have shown that nutrients separated from their food sources can act differently from what might be expected. Some studies of supplementary vitamins and minerals have also found adverse effects. Nutrition is not necessarily an area where more is better.

28

Antioxidants
– the hope and the hype

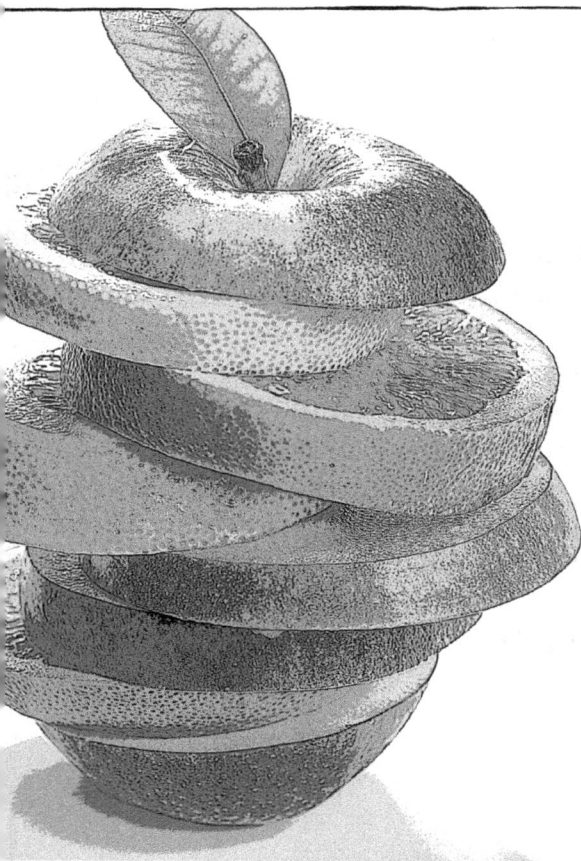

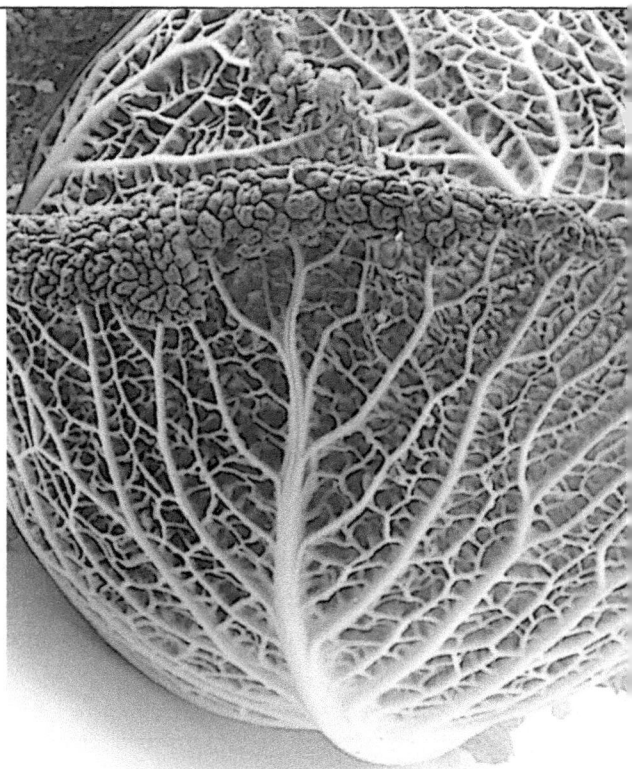

THE LIST OF FOODS promoted for their antioxidants continues to grow. Their antioxidant content is used to promote blueberries, plums and dried plums (prunes), cranberries, exotic berries, broccoli, tea, coffee and chocolate. Few people really understand what antioxidants do but the hype surrounding them has convinced many of us that they're 'good'. Indeed, advertisements in popular magazines plug antioxidants as great for preventing ageing, smoothing skin (via moisturisers and facial creams), as an essential part of 'detoxing', as aids to body-building (they're added to powdered soy and milk supplements), and in producing shiny healthy hair (check the shampoo bottle).

Most of the adulation for antioxidants has been fuelled by our youth-worshipping society's desire for anything that may stay the ravages of time. Most medical research into anti-ageing concentrates on normal blood pressure, clear arteries, healthy eyes and kidneys, sound teeth, a straight spine and dense bones, and a pancreas that produces appropriate quantities of insulin. For the majority of the public, however, interest in anti-ageing foods or treatments relates to avoiding sagging flesh, thinning hair and wrinkles, and the maintenance of sexual prowess. Whatever the perspective, there's a ready market for antioxidants when they are associated with preservation of youthfulness. Before swallowing the hype, it may be useful to know how much solid evidence backs many of the common beliefs.

What antioxidants do and don't do

Antioxidants play a vital role within foods and also within the body. In foods, exposure to oxygen can lead to oxidation reactions that turn apple flesh brown, make oils rancid and degrade the texture, flavour and nutrients in many products. Antioxidants prevent such reactions occurring.

Within the body, all oxygen-breathing animals, including humans, produce compounds called free radicals (more formally referred to by scientists as 'reactive oxygen species' or ROS) that cause disruption to cells. Fortunately, nature has given humans and other animals the ability to produce a range of antioxidants to deal with free radicals. There is some evidence suggesting that our production of antioxidants may decrease as we grow older. The hope is that antioxidants from foods may compensate for any shortfall in our own production. To keep this in perspective, however, we now know that free radicals are not eternal villains. New research shows that in appropriate quantities, free radicals are vital for the healthy functioning of body cells.

The ways in which antioxidants react in laboratory studies may also not be replicated in the body. Researchers deliberately generate large quantities of free radicals to induce damage so they can investigate the ways in which a particular antioxidant might alter their activity. These findings do not necessarily apply to the free radicals produced as a result of the body's normal use of oxygen. Any resemblance to the body's normal ageing process is also likely to be specific for particular cells, free radicals and antioxidants.

Within foods, the many different antioxidants have varying roles and effects. Some are more valuable than others so it is not valid to lump them all together and assume they are equally useful. Different testing methods to establish the level of antioxidants present in a food may also give an incomplete picture of the value of that food and its antioxidants. Tests usually rate the total antioxidant capacity of food, but different tests give different results and may not give a true indication of the potential value within the body.

Foods that are naturally rich in many hundreds of antioxidants include fruits, vegetables, extra virgin olive oil, wholegrains, nuts and tea. These foods are useful for many reasons, and some of their value almost certainly comes from specific antioxidants they contain. A few of the antioxidants in foods also happen to be vitamins, but most are not. And just as vitamin supplements don't always have the same beneficial function as the foods that contain them, research is also showing that isolated or purified antioxidants extracted from their natural sources may lose their usefulness. Taking extra antioxidants in specific foods or from supplements may have little effect on the cells in certain areas of the body.

Research on antioxidants and free radicals is usually done using fruit flies, nematodes (various species of roundworm) or, occasionally, mice. One recent study in nematodes found that inducing free radicals by mild treatment with oxidants acted as a signal to trigger changes in cells that reduced the effects of ageing. When the nematodes were given extra antioxidants, these effects were reversed and the worms' lifespan decreased. From this and other studies, some eminent researchers now stress that free radicals are a normal part of the body's stress response and, as such, may have beneficial effects. It is the *quantities* of free radicals produced and the type and quantity of antioxidants ingested that are important.

Of course, human ageing proceeds quite differently from the processes in fruit flies, nematodes and rodents, but we may need to hold the hype about antioxidants until we have results from well-designed human clinical trials. We also need to remember that attempts to flood the body with large quantities of extra antioxidants could be undesirable.

At this stage, no clinical trials have shown that chronic disease and ageing are due to over-production of free radicals. Nor have trials shown that consuming particular supplements or foods that have antioxidant activity will produce benefits. To add to the complexity, many of the compounds lauded as antioxidants, including various vitamins and minerals, have a wide range of roles within the body which may be quite separate from any antioxidant activity they show in test tubes.

Where are they found?

As well as the body's own production of antioxidants, literally hundreds of compounds with a variety of antioxidant effects are found in foods. The foods listed in the preceding section are all rich sources of antioxidants, although the different types found in them do not necessarily have the same biologic potency. Chocolate, herbs and spices, and coffee also contain antioxidants. Some vitamins, especially vitamins C and E and folate, can act as antioxidants, although this is not their sole role. The minerals zinc, copper and selenium are also antioxidants, but like many antioxidants, they can have an opposite pro-oxidant action if taken in large quantities. Clinical trials of various vitamins and minerals have not shown any significant benefits that could be ascribed to their antioxidant potential and some, such as beta carotene and vitamin E, have proven problematic. That said, new research into some of the 600 or more carotenoids in foods may reveal some benefits, especially for their potential roles in eye health.

Measuring antioxidants

It's not hard to find claims that blueberries or prunes or cranberries or pomegranates or acai berries or green tea or coffee or chocolate or even apples top the antioxidant table. The relevant response to these claims includes asking: Which antioxidants are we talking about and how were they measured? Which test was used for the measurement? Different tests will give different results and, even if the tests are accurate, may have little relevance to real life without knowing how well the particular antioxidants are absorbed or used or how much might be needed within the body. Without well-designed human studies, the tables of antioxidant levels have little meaning.

It's too soon to assume that antioxidants as a class are helpful or harmful for most aspects of human health. It's certainly premature to make exaggerated claims.

Types of antioxidants

CAROTENOIDS

More than 600 carotenoids have been isolated from fruits and vegetables. They are broadly divided into two major categories: the carotenes and the xanthophylls. Some of the more common ones and their sources are:

- alpha carotene (in carrots, pumpkins, sweet corn, oranges)
- beta carotene (in all brightly coloured fruits and vegetables, especially carrots, pumpkin, mango, pawpaw, broccoli, red capsicum, spinach, silverbeet)
- lycopene (in tomatoes, guava, pink grapefruit, watermelon)
- lutein (in spinach and other greens, egg yolk, red capsicum, pumpkin, mango, pawpaw, oranges, kiwi fruit, prunes, kumara, honeydew, plums, avocado)
- zeaxanthin (in spinach and other greens, egg yolk, red capsicum, pumpkin, oranges)
- cryptoxanthin (in mango, oranges, pawpaw, peaches, avocado, peas, kiwi fruit)
- astaxanthin (in prawns, salmon, lobster, crab).

33

For those interested in the range of antioxidant compounds and in polyphenols, a few basics may be useful. The terms 'antioxidant' and 'polyphenol' are sometimes used interchangeably and it is true that polyphenols are one type of antioxidant. Polyphenols can be subdivided into non-flavonoid polyphenols and flavonoids.

The *non-flavonoid polyphenols* include:

- lignans (in linseeds, sesame seeds, sunflower seeds, poppy seeds, berries, pears, oats and cruciferous vegetables)
- ellagitannins (in pomegranates and various berries)
- stilbenes (in red grapes, wine, blueberries and peanuts)
- xanthones (in the rind of mangosteen fruits, honeybush tea, St Johns Wort)
- phenolic acids (in coffee, spices, olive oil, capsicum, mango, walnuts, rhubarb, mustard, turmeric and whole grains)
- tyrosols (in extra virgin olive oil)
- coumarins (in citrus fruits and spices such as cinnamon).

Flavonoids can be subdivided into:

- flavanols (see below)
- anthocyanidins (in cherries, eggplant skin, red wine, berries, cherries)
- flavanones (in citrus fruit)
- flavones (in parsley, celery, citrus peel)
- flavonols (in tea, apples, onions, beans, berries, peas, grapes)
- flavonals (in plums, berries)
- isoflavonoids (in soy, alfalfa, peanuts, red clover).

Flavanols exist in various forms, including:

- catechins (in green tea, cocoa, dark chocolate, apples, red wine, lentils)
- proanthocyanidins (apples, cocoa, dark chocolate, grape seeds, red wine)
- thealanins (in tea) which can be further subdivided into theaflavins and thearubigins (both found in black and oolong teas).

A related range of antioxidants known as phenols is found in herbs such as rosemary, thyme, oregano, parsley and dill.

Artificial
sweeteners
– are they safe?

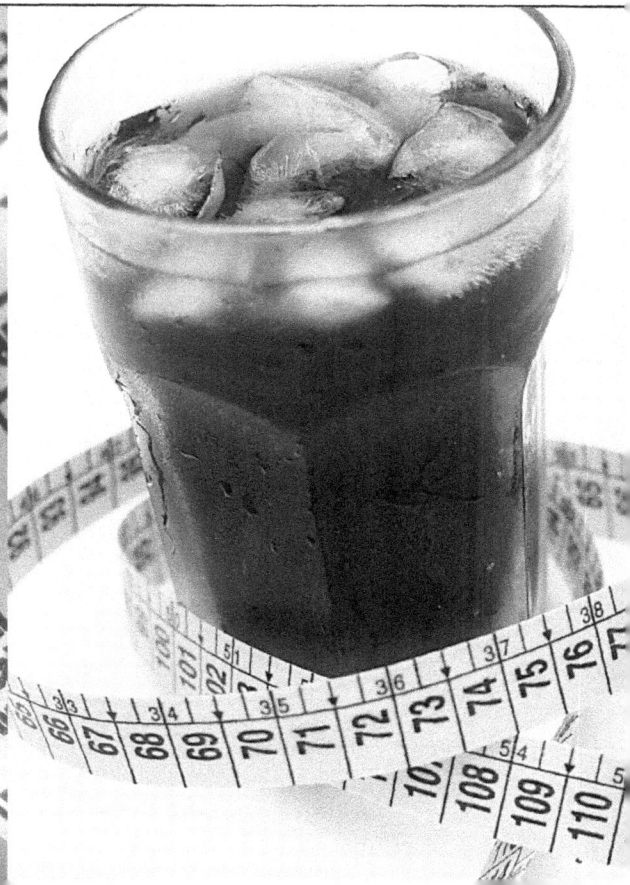

THE FIRST ARTIFICIAL SWEETENER, synthesised in 1879, was saccharin. It was widely used in the 1960s, but was banned in some countries after rat studies reported it was a possible carcinogen. About 50 per cent of the population also experience a bitter aftertaste from saccharin. Cyclamates were discovered next and found favour because many people found their flavour more appealing.

The range of artificial sweeteners continues to expand as food technologists discover new ways to isolate and synthesise intensely sweet compounds. Artificial sweeteners permitted in Australia (numbers 950–967) must be declared on food labels, along with the words 'artificially sweetened'. Those marketing these compounds prefer the term 'intense sweeteners', but since they are either man-ufactured or produced using sophisticated technology, the word 'artificial' is appropriate. That in itself is insufficient to damn them, however.

Any harm?

I avoid all artificial sweeteners because it seems absurd to use scarce energy resources to produce fake sugars (or fake fats) so that already overfed people can eat even more of the junk foods they are usually added to. I also harbour some ill-feeling towards some companies that own or produce some sweeteners. But even with my prejudices, I can't swallow all the stuff on many internet sites describing the unproven horrors of some sweeteners, especially aspartame. If the claims were even partly true, the millions of people who drink litres of diet soft drinks every day would be dead, or at least bed-bound. Each permitted artificial sweetener is also tested for safety, initially in animals. In these studies, rats or mice are given massive doses of the sweeteners to check for any harmful effects. This allows for an acceptable daily intake (ADI) to be established, with a large margin to account for potential indi-vidual variation in toxicity. Food authorities follow the principle that it is 'the dose that makes the poison', and in Australia, regular testing is conducted to gauge whether high consumers of any artificial sweetener are approaching the ADI.

Several laboratory studies have suggested that mixed drinks containing alcohol and diet cola may increase intoxication, especially in women. The problem arises because artificially sweetened drinks are absorbed faster than those containing sugar. Energy drinks that contain artificial sweeteners are particularly problematic when mixed with alcohol, as they are absorbed quickly and their high caffeine level can make drinkers unaware of how drunk they are.

Any use?

Many users of artificial sweeteners claim they can reduce their overall kilojoule intake by using foods containing artificial sweeteners, while many researchers believe that the continued use of intensely sweet foods is not only useless, but may work against weight loss.

Observational studies showing a correlation between the use of artificial sweeteners and obesity do not establish which came first, though – the use of sweeteners or the obesity. Several studies have reported that the use of artificial sweeteners increases hunger. Studies with animals have found that the sweeteners can stimulate cells within the intestine to release hormones that increase appetite. However, a recent comprehensive review of the effects of sweeteners has not shown consistent evidence to support an effect on appetite or subsequent food intake, or on the release of insulin within the body. At this stage, whether artificial sweeteners contribute to success or failure to lose weight is unclear. It may just be that using artificial sweeteners encourages people to feel free to consume other high-kilojoule foods. We have probably all seen someone adding a sweetener tablet to their cappuccino while indulging in a large cream cake!

With all studies on sweeteners, it is important to check the source of funding. Studies funded by companies with a vested interest in sugar sales tend to damn sweeteners, whereas studies funded by companies with a vested interest in increasing the use of artificial sweeteners may reach a different conclusion.

Approved sweeteners

ACESULPHAME K

Additive 950, acesulphame K, is 200 times as sweet as sugar. It is often used with other sweeteners in chewing gum, ice cream, confectionery and sweetened yoghurt. Safety tests have not revealed problems at the levels likely to be consumed.

ALITAME

Additive 956, alitame, is at least 2000 times as sweet as sugar. It is made from two amino acids (L-aspartic acid and D-alanine) and is permitted for use in drinks, jams, jellies, baked goods, custard and sweet spreads. No studies show harm at the very small levels used.

ASPARTAME

Additive 951, aspartame, is made up of derivatives of two amino acids, phenylalanine and aspartic acid. It is 200 times as sweet as sugar but can't be used in baked goods because the two amino acids break apart under heat and only taste sweet when they are together. Those with the rare genetic disorder phenylketonuria (PKU) cannot tolerate large quantities of phenylalanine and so food labels must warn of its presence. Aspartame is widely used in soft drinks, chewing gum, chocolate and confectionery and as a powdered sweetener.

Literally hundreds of internet sites damn aspartame, warning that it is a neurotoxin and chemical poison that can cause headaches, memory loss, chronic fatigue, brain lesions, seizures, mental retardation, depression, blindness and frequent epileptic attacks in pilots, Alzheimer's disease and multiple sclerosis. Some of the claims relate to the fact that aspartame breaks down in the body to produce methanol – a known toxin. However, the quantity of methanol produced is extremely small.

Part of the reason for the damnation of aspartame probably relates to the way it was first passed for consumption in the United States. Some (but not all) early studies showed potential problems with a high intake of aspartame. Its release was controversial, with the head of the US Food and Drug Administration allegedly sacked (in 1981) after he refused to approve it. His successor passed regulations permitting aspartame and later accepted a job with the makers of the sweetener. Similar 'revolving-door' relationships have been apparent with approvals for some genetically modified products from the same company and this, naturally, gives rise to suspicion.

Problems arose again in 1992 when a study suggested that aspartame could cause problems for children who suffered with a particular type of brain seizure. Subsequent studies by an independent group did not confirm the findings. Another study in 2006 reported that aspartame could increase cancer in rats. European investigators re-examined all the evidence, giving aspartame a clean bill of health at the current low levels set for the ADI. Official Australian surveys show that the average person who uses products sweetened with aspartame consumes quantities equivalent to 6 per cent of the ADI, with even the heaviest consumers reaching only 15 per cent of the ADI.

There is no need for anyone to use aspartame, and that includes those who are overweight or have diabetes. Many of the products containing it are junk foods. However, the outrage it provokes is not backed by scientific evidence and the same emails that warn of 'new' evidence have been released regularly for over 25 years.

CYCLAMATES

Additive 952 (referring to both sodium cyclamate and calcium cyclamate) was first made in 1937; it was banned for many years in the US and the UK for fear it could lead to bladder cancer. Further studies cleared it of suspicion in quantities below the ADI. Cyclamates are 40 times as sweet as sugar and widely used in cordials and soft drinks. Permitted levels in cordials have recently been reduced by half in Australia because the top 5 per cent of cordial drinkers were consuming quantities close to the ADI.

ERYTHRITOL

Additive 968, erythritol, is made from glucose that has been treated with a yeast that converts it to a form that cannot be digested in the intestine. It is less sweet than sugar (about 70 per cent of the sweetness) and most of it is excreted unchanged. It contributes only 1 kJ/g and can be used to replace up to 10 per cent of the sugar in cakes; it is also

39

used in chocolates, confectionery, pickles, beverages and frozen desserts. There is no evidence of harm at this stage.

ISOMALT

Additive 953, isomalt, is made from sugar beet and is as sweet as sugar but provides only half the kilojoules. It also functions as a bulking agent and a humectant to keep foods moist. It is broken down in the body to form glucose, sorbitol and mannitol. A high intake of sorbitol and mannitol can cause diarrhoea and wind. It is used in ice cream, cakes and confectionery, and recent reports show that it is used by the bacteria that cause erosion of tooth enamel. Dentists therefore warn that lollies and cough drops containing isomalt are a dental hazard.

LACTITOL

Additive 966, lactitol, is made from lactose, the sugar in milk. It has only 40 per cent of the sweetness of sugar and half the kilojoules of sugar, and is usually used with more concentrated sweeteners. Like all sugar alcohols, it is only partly digested in the small intestine, then passes to the large intestine where it has a laxative effect and causes wind. It is used in confectionery, frozen desserts, chocolate, cakes, pickles and dressings, drinks, sauces and sports foods.

MALTITOL

Additive 965, maltitol, is made from malted grains and functions as a sweetener, humectant and emulsifier. It has about three-quarters of the sweetness of sugar and is used with other, more concentrated sweeteners. Like other sugar alcohols, it can have a laxative effect and cause wind. It is used in chewing gum, confectionery, ice cream and chocolate.

NEOTAME

Additive 961, neotame, is made from the same two amino acids used to make aspartame – aspartic acid and phenylalanine – but the amino acids are joined with a stronger bond than in aspartame so that this sweetener is stable for use in cakes and baked goods. It is not broken down to its component amino acids in the body, but is excreted. No harmful effects have been identified in safety tests.

SACCHARIN

Additive 954, saccharin, is made from by-products of coal and is 200–500 times as sweet as sugar. It is not digested in the body and is excreted by the kidneys. In 1977, saccharin was banned in the United States after Canadian researchers found it caused bladder cancer in rats. Following an outcry from the general public, diabetic associations and the soft drink industry, the substance was re-examined, with new studies showing it did not cause bladder cancer in mice and that people with diabetes who used saccharin for some years had no increased risk of bladder cancer. This led to its removal from the Report on Carcinogens and it was permitted in the US with a warning label. Australia has always permitted saccharin as a sweetener as authorities consider it would be difficult to consume enough to create a hazard.

STEVIA

Additive 960, stevia, is made from the plant *Stevia rebaudiana* (a member of the chrysanthemum family) and was approved for use in Australia in 2008. It is 250 times as sweet as sugar and is sold as a 'smart' tabletop sweetener, mixed with raw or white sugar. Its taste has hints of treacle and licorice. Tests show that stevia is safe in the quantities likely to be consumed. Suspicion arose in the United States when stevia was approved as a 'midnight gift' to the soft drink industry on the departure of President George W. Bush. It is favoured by those who want more natural products.

SUCRALOSE

Additive 955, sucralose, is 600 times as sweet as sugar and is made by replacing some of the atoms in sugar with chlorine. Claims this organochloride is 'natural' because it is made from sugar stretch credulity, but regulatory authorities in many parts of the world assess it as safe. The structure of sucralose means it can't be broken down by enzymes in the intestine, so it passes through the intestine without contributing kilojoules. It is stable under heat and can be used in cakes, biscuits and other baked goods as well as breakfast cereals, confectionery and sweet sauces. It is sold as the tabletop sweetener Splenda, and is often listed by this name in recipes. No evidence of any harmful properties has yet emerged, although some other organochlorides can be toxic.

THAUMATIN

Additive 957, thaumatin, is 2000 times as sweet as sugar. It is extracted from the fruit of the West African plant *Thaumatococcus danielli*, and has a delayed sweet flavour. It is most likely to be used in fruit juices, soft drinks and confectionery, but its extreme sweetness is a barrier to widespread use in food manufacturing. It is marketed in some countries as Talin.

XYLITOL

Additive 967, xylitol, occurs naturally in fruits and vegetables, especially in strawberries, raspberries and cauliflower. It has similar degree of sweetness to sugar, but only half the kilojoules because it is only partly digested in the small intestine with the residue passing to the large intestine. Large quantities lead to diarrhoea and wind. Xylitol has some protective effects on tooth enamel because it blocks the uptake of glucose by the bacteria that cause tooth decay. It can also be heated or frozen without losing its sweet taste. It is used in chewing gum, confectionery, frozen desserts, low-kilojoule products and baked goods.

Beans
and other
legumes
– ticking all the boxes

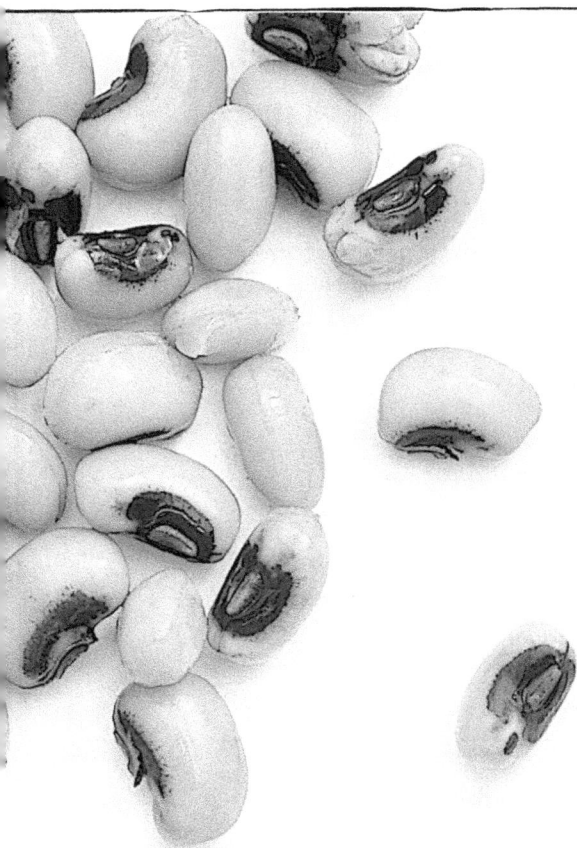

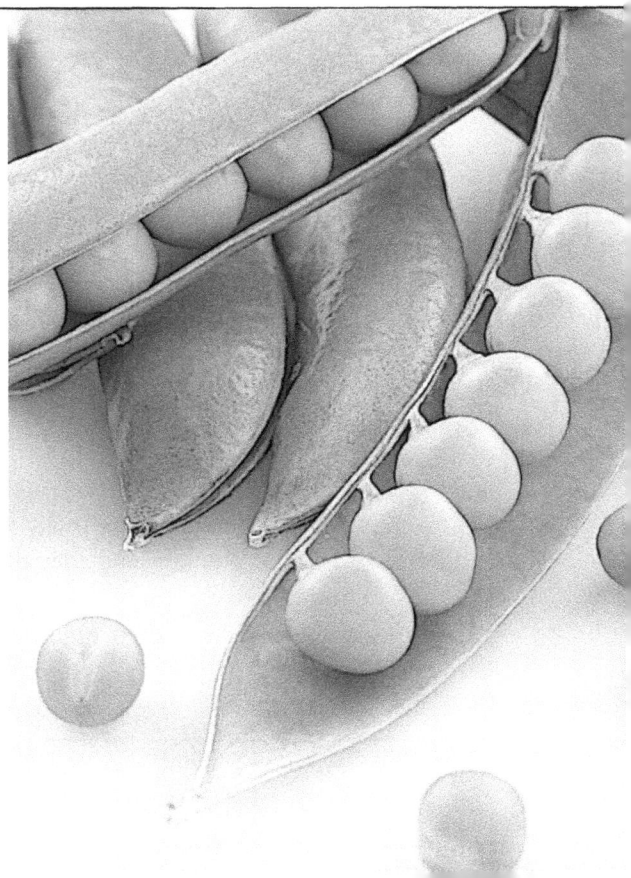

FOR ANY FOOD TO GET MY FULL APPROVAL, it must meet three criteria: it must taste good; it must *be* good for you; and it must create minimal environmental damage in its growth and preparation. Legumes (dried peas and beans) tick all three boxes. Add the fact that they are economical and you realise why dried beans and peas feature in most of the world's great cuisines. People in Mediterranean and Middle Eastern countries especially have long known the joys and benefits of legumes.

Apart from traditional vegetarians, Australians have been slow to make great use of legumes, although products such as hummus are now used widely. Nutritionists are hopeful that the popularity of many dishes with legumes will grow so that these highly nutritious foods take a more important role in the diet.

The nutritional virtues

Legumes are excellent sources of:

- protein, ranging from 15–18 g/cup of cooked legumes
- dietary fibre, including soluble and insoluble types and ranging from 6–14 g/cup cooked
- minerals such as iron and zinc
- vitamins of the B complex, especially thiamin (B1), niacin (B3), pyridoxine (B6), folate, biotin and pantothenic acid, and some vitamin E
- carbohydrate in a form that is digested and absorbed slowly, thus avoiding any rise in blood glucose levels
- fat content is mostly low, with the notable exception of soy beans which are high in polyunsaturated fatty acids, including both omega 6 (mainly as linoleic acid) and omega 3 (alpha-linolenic acid or ALA)
- phytonutrients are also high and include some compounds that act as antioxidants and some with anti-cancer activity.

Canned beans

When canned, beans retain their nutrients well. If they are canned in water, you can consider them as equivalent in nutritional value to home-cooked beans. Some manufacturers add salt and this detracts somewhat from their high nutritional status, but they are still a useful and nutritious product. Draining and rinsing them will decrease the salt content. Canned baked beans (usually haricot beans) are a handy quick meal with better nutritional value than, say, most take-away foods. The highest rating goes to brands without added salt.

Which legume?

CHICK PEAS

If you don't regularly use legumes, start with chick peas. Their firm texture and almost nutty flavour appeals to most people – even those who think they don't like beans. Mediterranean and Middle Eastern cuisines have long valued chick peas (sometimes called garbanzos or ceci). Made into hummus, or served with couscous, added to soups, stews and salads, chick peas are a constant feature of the healthy diets of these regions. Chick peas are also popular in India, where they are traditionally combined with spices and onions to make nutritious and delicious curries. Roasted spiced chick peas make a great pre-dinner snack.

Roast cooked chick peas in a moderate oven for 20–30 minutes. Toss with chilli powder, freshly ground pepper and dried parsley flakes.

SPICED CHICK PEAS

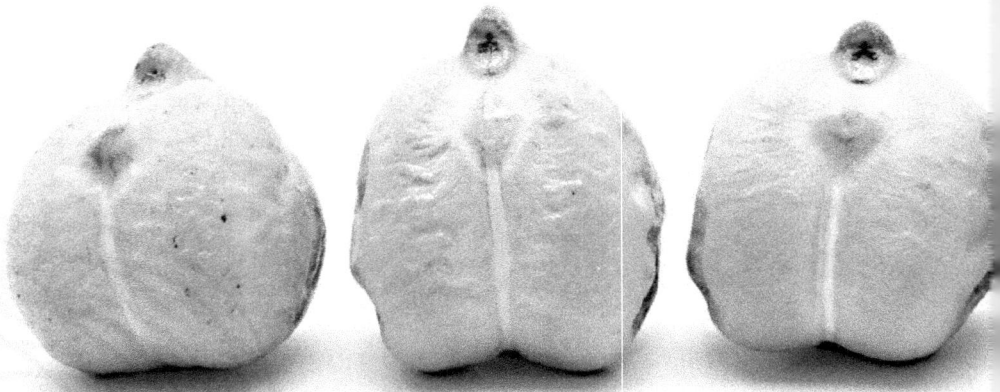

HUMMUS

1–2 cups cooked or canned, drained chick peas

1–2 cloves crushed garlic

juice of 1 lemon

1–2 tablespoons tahini (sesame seed paste)

Blend chick peas with garlic, lemon juice, tahini and enough of the cooking water or canned liquid to form a thick paste.

BLACK-EYED BEANS

These small, white, kidney-shaped beans have a black spot at the sprouting point and are also known as black-eyed peas, cow peas or black-eyed Susans. Their thin skin means they cook faster than many other beans and they do not need to be soaked. Although they originated in Africa, they are widely used in Middle Eastern, Indian and Greek cookery.

BORLOTTI BEANS

Also known as Roman, cranberry, saluggia or rosecoco beans, these plump and pretty beans are usually speckled pink, but may also be beige or brown. Their smooth texture and slightly ham-like flavour make them popular in soups and Italian dishes. Use borlotti beans in recipes that call for pinto beans when pinto beans are unavailable.

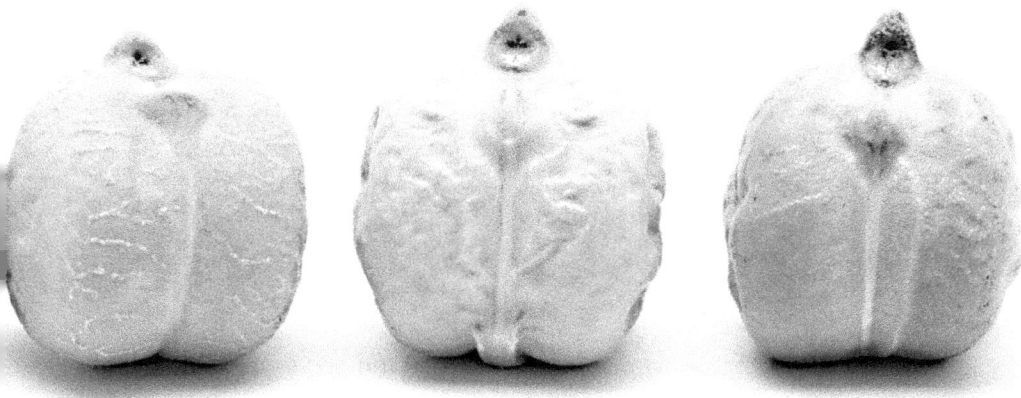

HARICOT BEANS

These small white oval-shaped beans are mainly used for canned baked beans. They're also known as navy beans and are widely used in the Middle East and the Mediterranean. Canned baked beans are nutritious and make a quick snack-type meal. Check the label and choose a brand with the lowest sodium content.

KIDNEY BEANS

Red kidney beans are most common, but they also come in brown, black and white forms. Originally from the West Indies, kidney beans are now used throughout the world, especially in South America's famous chilli con carne. Canned kidney beans are convenient and nutritious, and are excellent in a bean soup or as a salad, tossed with extra virgin olive oil, lemon zest and lots of chopped flat leaf parsley.

LENTILS

One of the first legumes to be cultivated, lentils rate several mentions in the Old Testament. Red, green and brown lentils are widely used in India, Middle Eastern countries and parts of Eastern Europe; France is famous for the high-quality blue-grey Puy lentil. Puy lentils are now grown in Australia and although they are more expensive than other lentils, the cost per serve is still very modest in comparison with the meat they can replace. Green lentils need soaking before cooking, but red and brown split lentils and the blue-grey variety can

47

simply be simmered for less than 30 minutes. Mashed lentils, flavoured with plenty of chopped herbs and bound with a beaten egg and fresh breadcrumbs, can be made into lentil burgers. Or you can make dhal, the lentil purée that is a major source of protein in India. Lentils are also great in soups, used to 'extend' casseroles, and cooked with lamb shanks.

LIMA BEANS

These large butter beans originated in Peru and are used as young fresh green beans (with a high content of vitamin C) or in the more mature, larger dried form. They are widely used in soups and casseroles.

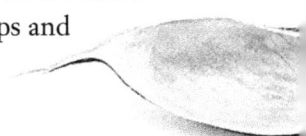

MUNG BEANS

Native to India, tiny green mung beans, also called green gram, are popular throughout Asia. The beans do not need to be soaked and can be cooked and eaten whole or ground into flour for use in pancakes. Mostly, however, they are available as the familiar plump sprouts which are ideal in salads or used in Asian soups such as laksa. Bean sprouts do not need to be cooked. When you make laksa, just place the fresh sprouts into the bowl and pour the hot laksa over them.

SOY BEANS

Probably one of the most important food crops throughout the world, the small, oval, light brown soy bean originated in China and has been a staple food throughout Asia for over 5000 years. Soy beans are also made into tofu and the fermented tempeh, soy beverages, soy flour and soy sauce. Soy sauce, however, does not retain the valuable nutrients of the soy bean, and even salt-reduced varieties are high in sodium. Soy protein can also be spun into fibres and used in meat substitutes. Unlike most legumes, soy beans contain fat, with about 17 g fat per 100 g of beans. The fat is a healthy polyunsaturated kind.

Fresh green soy beans, known as edamame, are popular in Japan and make a healthy snack. Edamame are available frozen in Asian groceries. Like chick peas, dried cooked soy beans can be roasted to make a healthy snack.

48

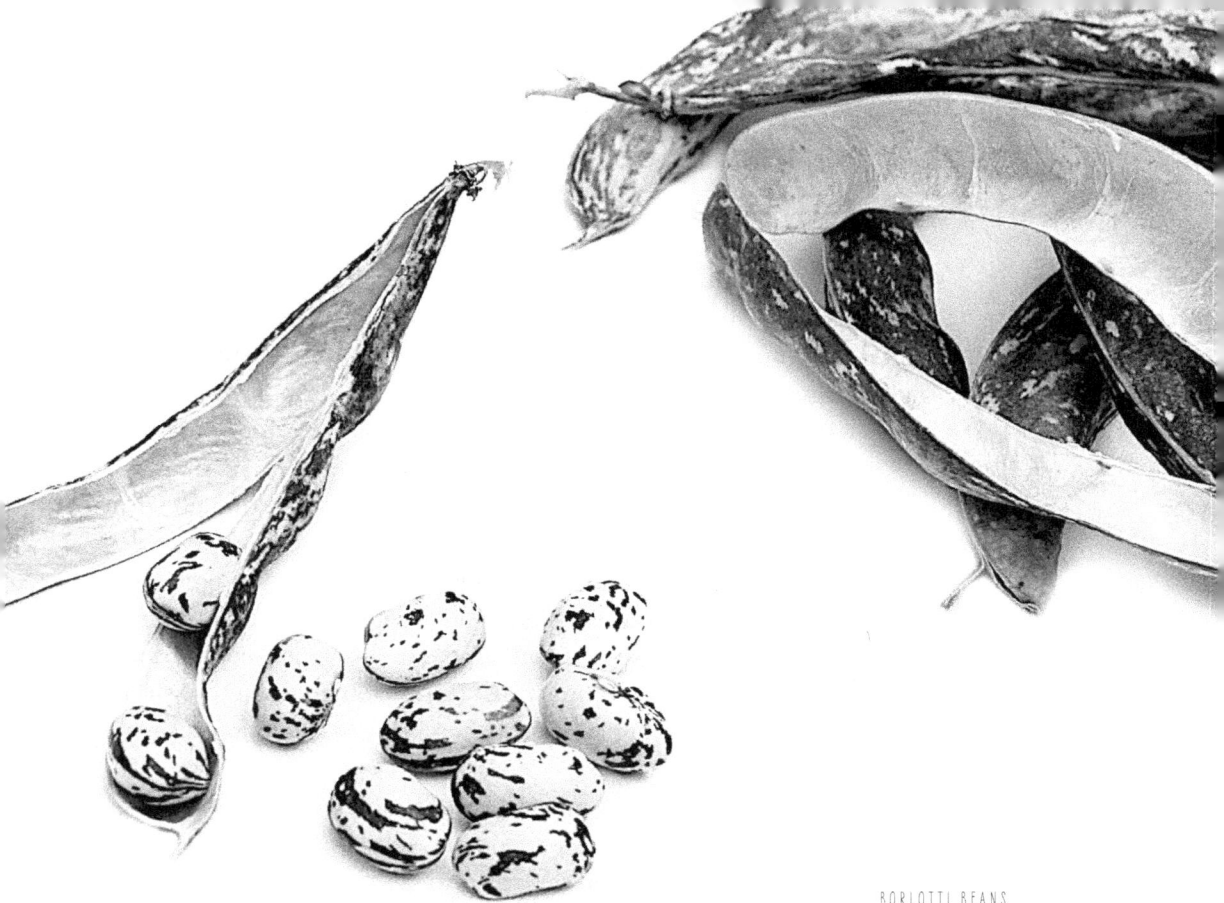

BORLOTTI BEANS

OTHER LEGUMES

Many other highly nutritious legumes are available, including:

- aduki (or adzuki or feijao), used in candied bean cakes
- black gram (or urad), often ground into flour for flatbreads
- cannellini, from Argentina, closely related to haricot beans
- fava beans, usually consumed fresh as broad beans
- ful medames, a small round brown bean popular in Egypt and the Middle East
- lupins, which were once considered inedible because of their high content of toxic alkaloids, are now bred without these hazardous compounds and often ground into flour for use in breads, noodles and making miso
- pigeon peas, also known as red gram, congo peas, gungar or arhar, and mostly sold as split peas
- pinto beans, creamy beans with pink speckles, used in Mexican dishes
- tepary beans, beige in colour and related to haricot beans, used in Central American cuisines.

49

Cooking legumes

Lentils and black eyed beans do not need to be soaked before cooking, but most other legumes require soaking for several hours. Leave them soaking overnight (in summer, preferably in the refrigerator to prevent fermentation). After soaking, pour off the water, cover with fresh water and simmer until the beans are tender. A faster method is to place legumes into a saucepan, cover with water, bring to the boil, top with a close fitting lid and turn the heat off. Stand for one hour, pour off the soaking water, cover with fresh water and simmer until tender. Most beans cook in an hour or so, although soy beans need at least two hours to become tender. You can cook a big pot of legumes that can be frozen in smaller portions ready for quick use. One point to note: any acidic ingredients stop beans softening, so always pre-cook dried beans (including lentils) before adding them to dishes containing vinegar, lemon juice or acidic foods such as tomatoes.

Do not eat raw dried legumes, especially kidney beans, as they contain substances called lectins that can destroy vitamins and damage cells, especially in the liver and kidneys. Lectins are destroyed by cooking.

Wind fears

Eating legumes increases the production of gases in the colon. This may be a social problem in many cultures, but it is not a medical one. Legumes contain sugars that are not digested in the small intestine. These pass to the colon where 'good' bacteria feast on them and dietary fibre from the beans. While enjoying their sweet meal, the bacteria produce gas – and short chain fatty acids that help protect the bowel against cancer. Soaking legumes and discarding the soaking water reduces the sugar content and the gas production.

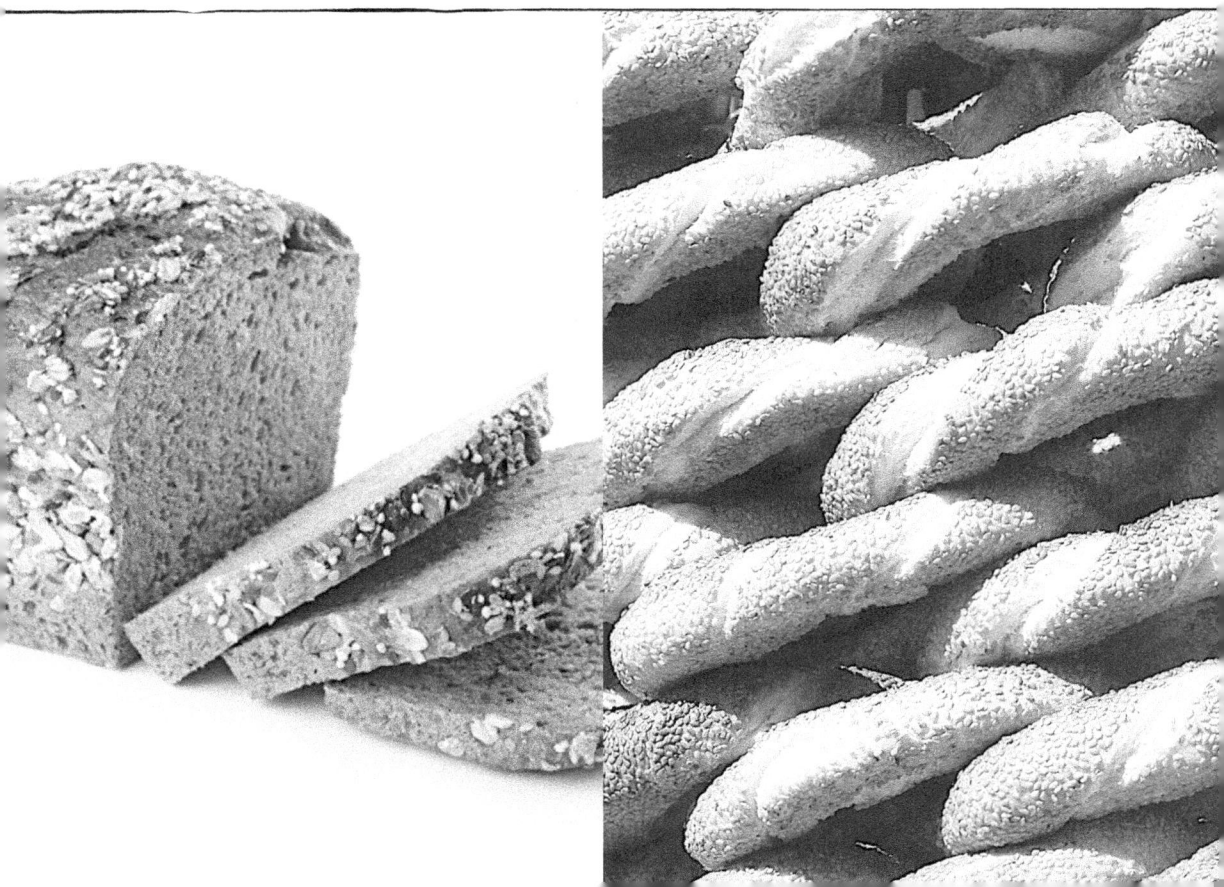

Bread

THOUSANDS OF YEARS AGO, the leavened and unleavened flat-breads enjoyed in countries of the Middle East, southern India, China, and many of the countries around the Mediterranean, including Italy and the countries of North Africa, became part of the daily diet. The grains ground to make these breads included wheat, rye, corn, barley, oats, sorghum, rice and buckwheat. Potatoes, chick peas, lentils and various beans were also ground into flour and used in traditional flat-breads. In many areas where fuels were and still are scarce, flatbreads remain popular because they cook quickly. Those who suffer adverse reactions to the gluten in wheat, rye and barley are leading a revival in popularity of many of the other gluten-free grains and flours.

Who eats bread?

Bread remains an integral part of every meal in many parts of the world, especially in Mediterranean and Middle Eastern countries. Europeans have much more respect for bread than people in Australia, the United Kingdom or the United States. Go to France and you can't miss the aroma of the traditional baguette. The Italians mop up olive oil and food juices with quality breads still made in the traditional slow-rising way. Germans prefer heavy rye breads, with lighter rye loaves popular in Scandinavian countries.

Australian bread consumption has almost halved over the last 50 years. Toast was once traditional at breakfast and almost everyone took sand-wiches or bread rolls to school or work for lunch. Cereals or croissants or skipping breakfast altogether have decreased bread consumption at breakfast and many fast foods now compete for lunchtime favour. Bread consumption has also fallen as people have jumped on the low-carb bandwagon. Somewhat ironically, as bread intake goes down, obesity rises.

The advantages of bread

TASTE

People of all ages enjoy bread, whether as a fresh loaf or toasted. It's fun to make and the smell of a freshly baked loaf makes most people's mouths water.

52

Contrary to popular belief, bread is much more than carbohydrate. The starchy carbs in bread come with dietary fibre, protein (bread has 8–12 per cent protein, which is about half the level of meat), B complex vitamins (especially thiamin and folate – both of which are added to bread flour), and some valuable minerals (including magnesium, iron and calcium). Since 2009, it's also been mandatory for Australian bread makers to use iodised salt and this now makes bread a major source of iodine. People who consume bread plus other foods containing iodine (milk, seafood) should now obtain adequate quantities from foods, although pregnant women still need an iodine supplement. Wholemeal and wholegrain breads have the highest levels of dietary fibre, vitamins and minerals.

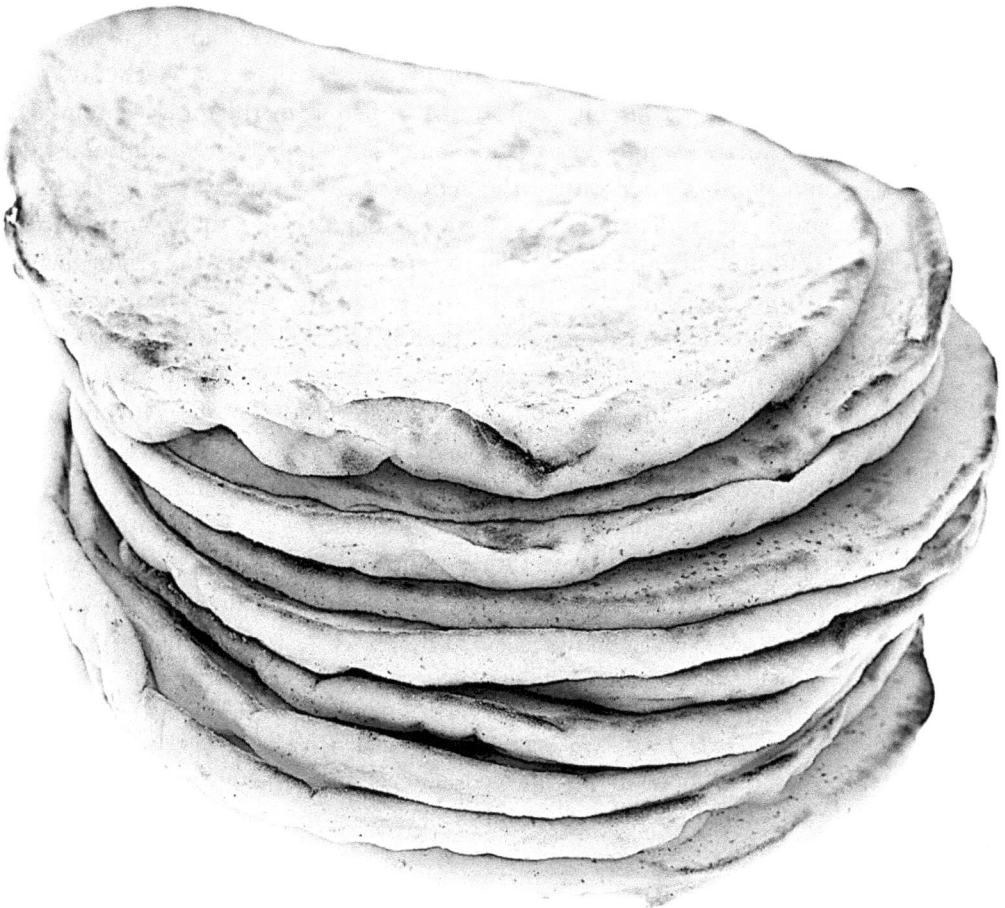

Most breads are filling, especially those that include whole grains. Studies show that when we take in kilojoules from a sweet drink (including fruit juice), we are unlikely to reduce the quantity of other foods consumed. However, bread 'sticks to the ribs' and generally means we eat less of something else. Breads that have more dietary fibre or a low glycaemic index (GI) are digested more slowly and are more filling, with wholegrain and sourdough breads usually being the most filling.

CONVENIENCE

Bread keeps well, can be frozen, is easy to transport, popular with people of all ages, can be toasted, makes a great snack and comes in many varieties, including many that are super healthy.

What does bread contain?

The only ingredients necessary for making bread are flour, usually from wheat with a higher protein content than the wheat used to make cake or biscuit flour; and fortified with thiamin (vitamin B1) and folate; water; yeast and some salt, added to retain moisture and stabilise and control the action of the yeast. Some breads from small or independent bakeries contain only these ingredients. Traditionally, these ingredients are combined in the right proportions, the dough is kneaded and left to rise over an hour or two – or longer for sourdough – and then it is 'knocked' down, formed into loaves and allowed to rise again before being baked. Bread made by this method has a low glycaemic index, whatever kind of flour it contains.

Modern mass-produced packaged breads usually contain a variety of other ingredients, including rapid dough risers, so the bread dough is mixed by machine and then allowed to rise over a few minutes before being shaped into loaves. Other additives may include:

- *sugar*, added in small quantities (2–4 g/loaf) as food for the yeast
- *fat*, which makes bread soft and so extends its life; fats containing trans fat are used in some breads, but the quantity per slice is small
- *emulsifiers* to interact with the starches to maintain a soft crumb
- *bread improver* – often ascorbic acid (vitamin C), which feeds the yeast
- *preservatives*, such as propionic acid to prevent mould (often added only in

54

hot weather); some people claim that propionic acid causes adverse reactions including rashes and temper tantrums; those who think it may cause problems can check the ingredient list and avoid additive 280

- *dough 'improvers'* or enzymes, which may include ascorbic acid (vitamin C) to change the action of the gluten in the flour, or rapid dough risers such as ammonium chloride, phosphates and calcium salts.

Glycaemic index and bread

The rapid dough risers used in modern mass-production reduce the time needed to make a loaf of bread but also change the nature of the starch granules in the loaf. When these breads are eaten, their starches are digested much more quickly than the starches in traditionally made bread, giving the modern loaf a higher glycaemic index (GI). This applies to bread made using both white and wholemeal flours; if the whole grains are stoneground and the bread contains bits of grain, this slows down the digestive process and reduces the GI.

Types of bread

WHOLEMEAL

Wholemeal breads should contain ground whole wheat. Most wholemeal bread in Australia is made (quite legally) from white flour combined with wheat bran and wheat germ, added in the same proportions as in the original grain. All wholemeal breads have a high content of dietary fibre, minerals and vitamins, but standard loaves made from recombined grain usually have a higher GI than breads made from more traditionally ground flour. Smooth wholemeal breads are useful for small children and some elderly people who prefer to avoid 'bits' in their bread.

WHOLEGRAIN

Wholegrain breads are made from the whole wheat grain, and the flour may be coarsely or finely ground. Wholegrain breads have similar nutrient levels to wholemeal bread, but are digested more slowly and have a lower GI.

55

MIXED GRAIN

Mixed grain (also called multigrain) breads are made from white flour with added pieces of soaked whole grains. Their nutritional value is half way between white and wholemeal but the presence of 'bits' gives these loaves a lower GI than smooth wholemeal.

SEEDED

Seeded breads are usually wholemeal or wholegrain loaves with added linseeds (also called flaxseeds), sunflower, poppy and sesame seeds. These seeds contribute omega 3 fats (mainly from linseeds) and vitamin E. Most are also high in dietary fibre and so are useful for those who may suffer from constipation.

WHITE

White breads are made from wheat grain that has had the bran and germ removed. Australian wheats are high in nutrients so white breads retain significant quantities of nutrients and some dietary fibre. In general, white bread has just under half the fibre content of wholemeal bread.

RYE

Rye breads usually combine wheat and rye flours. Rye flour has a little less gluten than wheat flour and this gives the bread a denser texture. Light rye may have 30 per cent rye flour and 70 per cent white wheat flour, whereas heavier German-style breads are 60–100 per cent rye. The level of dietary fibre and nutrients varies according to the amount of white flour added. Check the ingredient list on the label.

SOURDOUGH

Sourdough breads are made with natural (also called 'wild') yeasts, although some may also contain added regular baker's yeast. The dough is usually left to ferment over many hours; this provides the familiar flavour and also ensures that all sourdough loaves (white or wholegrain) have a low GI.

RAISIN/FRUIT

Raisin and fruit breads make a healthy snack food and are ideal for toasting. A slice of lightly buttered raisin toast has more nutrients and far fewer kilojoules than a slice of cake or a couple of biscuits.

PITA/FLATBREAD

Pitas, pide (or Turkish bread) and flatbreads such as lavash may or may not include yeast. Some are made from white flour, others from wholemeal. Check the ingredient list on individual products.

FOCACCIA

Focaccia is a moist, flat, yeasted Italian bread with the dough brushed with olive oil and topped with sea salt flakes and other ingredients such as black olives, onion or herbs. It has a higher salt and fat content than most breads, although the fat content can be readily accommodated by forgoing the use of a spread.

GLUTEN-FREE

Gluten-free breads, made without wheat, rye, barley or oat flour, usually contain a mixture of flours chosen from potato, corn, millet, quinoa, sorghum, buckwheat, rice or legumes such as soy. Since gluten provides the crust and texture of bread, gluten-free loaves are usually heavier and more scone-like than regular bread. The nutritional value varies with the grains used.

Is bread fattening?

Whether or not any food is fattening depends on the quantity consumed in relation to the person's needs. A typical 40 g slice of bread has about 400 kJ, which is about the same as an average 175 g apple. Bread is rarely a problem in the day's total intake, especially as it is fairly filling and many varieties are a good source of nutrients. The spreads added to bread can contribute more kilojoules than the bread itself, although this depends on the quantity used. To put the kilojoules in bread into perspective, most people who need to lose weight need to confine their daily kilojoule intake to about 6500 kJ. That can easily accommodate several slices of bread, as long as a frugal quantity of spread is used. It is worth noting that the weight of a slice of ready-sliced bread has increased over the years from about 28 g to 40 g. Some toast slices may be even more.

Breakfast
cereals
– a good start to the day?

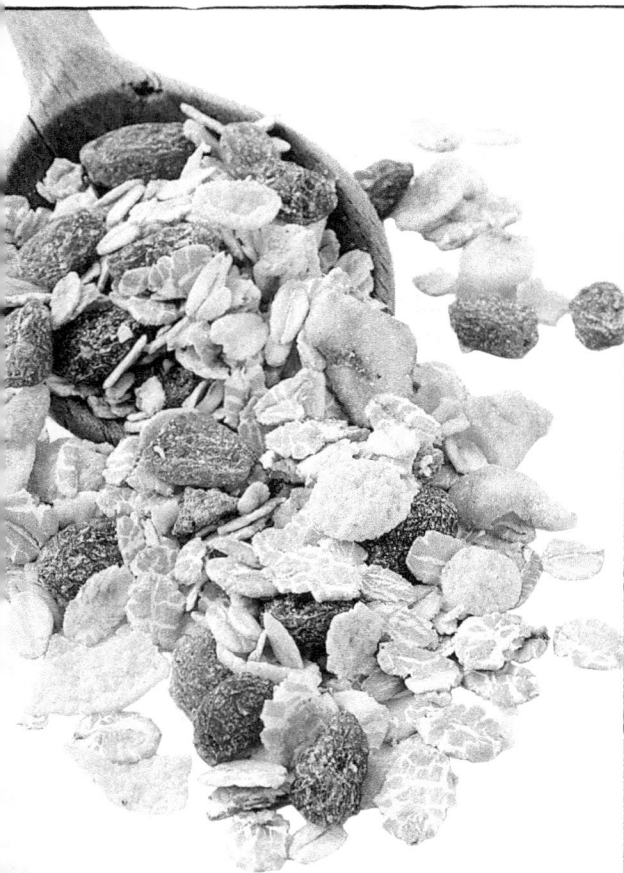

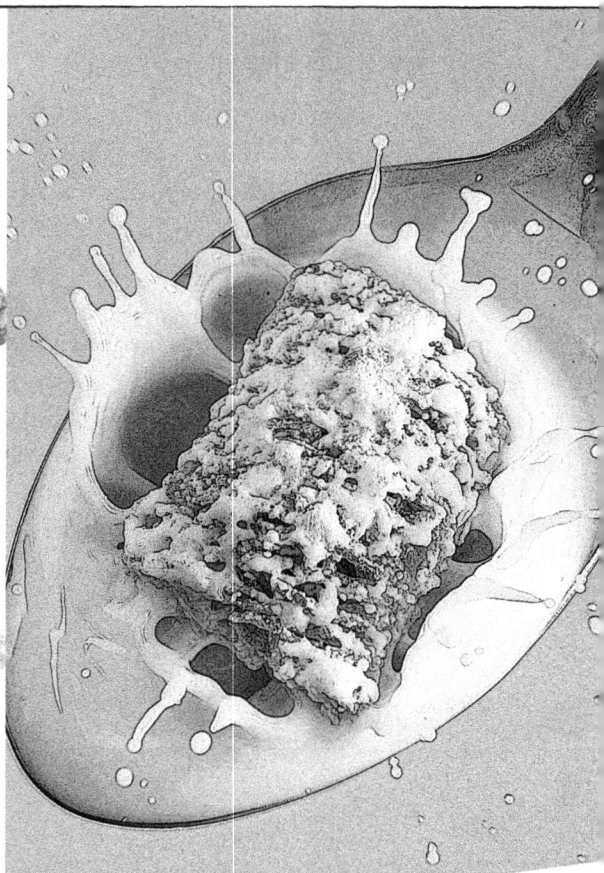

OVERNIGHT, THE BODY'S METABOLIC RATE SLOWS. Just getting up and moving about raises it somewhat, but eating breakfast gets the body going. There is no ideal food for breakfast, but cereals are commonly consumed in Australia.

Walking down the breakfast cereal aisle, it's easy to believe that Australians are the world's largest consumers of breakfast cereals. Most supermarkets stock about 150 different cereal products plus a wide range of breakfast cereal bars. Some breakfast cereals are made from whole grains, and may be highly nutritious products with added dried fruit, nuts and seeds contributing dietary fibre, protein, minerals and vitamins. Other highly processed puffed, popped or extruded products have so few remaining nutrients that manufacturers add vitamins and minerals. The flavour is also destroyed by such processing, so sugar is added, in amounts that range from as little as 1 per cent in some products up to half the product. Most processed breakfast cereal products are around one-third sugar. Even though sugar is usually cheaper than grains, the price usually rises in line with the sugar content. Many people are surprised that salt is also added, presumably to add flavour and tone down the sugar. Products designed to appeal to children may also have added chocolate flavouring and colourings.

Top of the range

The most nutritious breakfast cereals include rolled oats or oatmeal, wheatmeal or mixed-grain porridges, and some mueslis. Wheat germ is particularly high in nutrients and adding 2 tablespoons to other cereals will increase the overall value of your breakfast. Wholewheat breakfast biscuits and high-fibre mixed cereals, often with added dried fruits, are also healthy choices.

Muesli can vary from a top quality product to one that is nutritionally equivalent to a bowl of broken up sweet biscuits. Check the ingredient list, especially with toasted mueslis, which may contain a lot of added sugar and fat. Better quality muesli containing nuts, seeds and dried fruit usually costs more. It may be cheaper to make your own and you can vary the ingredients to suit your budget and taste. Toasting the oats and nuts intensifies their flavour.

TOASTED
MUESLI

1 kg rolled oats

100 g flaked almonds

1/4 cup sesame seeds or linseeds

1/2 cup flaked coconut*

100 g pepitas

100 g sunflower seeds

1 cup wheat germ

1 cup chopped dried apricots

1 cup sultanas

1/2 cup craisins

1. Preheat oven to 180°C. Spread oats on two ungreased oven trays and bake for 8–10 minutes, stirring several times until the oats are golden brown (take care they don't burn). Tip into a large bowl and allow to cool.

2. Toast almonds and sesame seeds by the same method, watching carefully as they take only 2–3 minutes. Set aside to cool. (Do not toast linseeds.)

3. Toast coconut in the same way, leaving it in the oven for a maximum of 1–2 minutes only (it burns easily). Cool.

4. Combine all ingredients and store in an airtight container.

Makes about 30 × 60 g serves

* Coconut adds 0.7 g saturated fat/serve. This is a small quantity, but omit if desired.

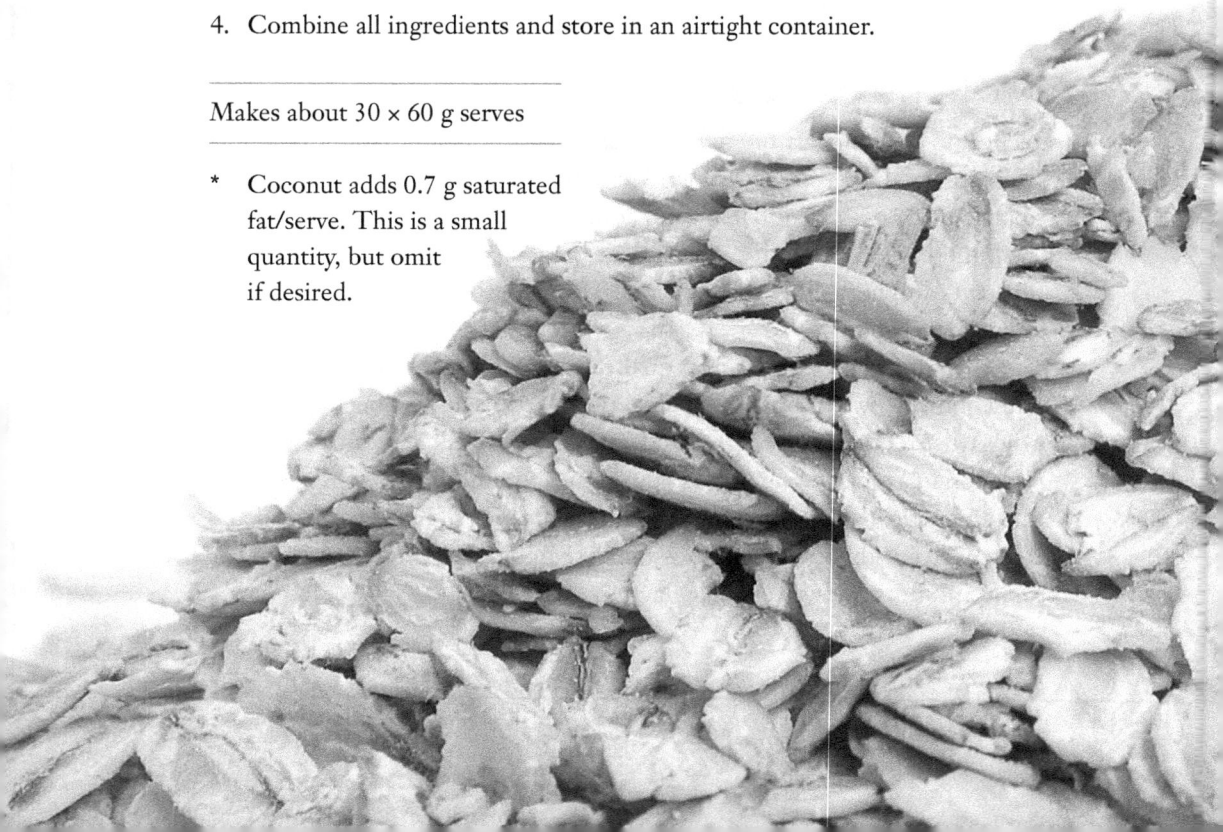

Scraping the sugar barrel

The more sugar a product contains, the lower its possible content of whole grains. The nutrition information panel will list all sugars in the product, including those that are naturally present in dried fruit. To get some idea of the added sugar content, check the ingredient list, where the contents must be listed in descending order of prominence. Be aware, however, that some manufacturers use several forms of sugar (perhaps selected from raw sugar, honey, maltose, glucose, fructose) to avoid having sugar top the ingredient list. If a product is 50 per cent sugar and 48 per cent rice, the ingredients should be listed as sugar, rice, then salt, colouring, etc. However, if the manufacturer uses 25 per cent each of two *different* sugars, the rice will be listed as the major ingredient. If you want cereal rather than sugar, avoid products with several types of sugar in the ingredient list.

Most high sugar products have little dietary fibre, although some manufacturers are now adding a limited quantity of finely milled whole grains to the product so they can announce this on the front of the pack. Manufacturers claim that pre-sweetening products means that children will not need to add sugar. This ignores the fact that few children would be permitted to add enough sugar to a cereal to make up more than half the bowl.

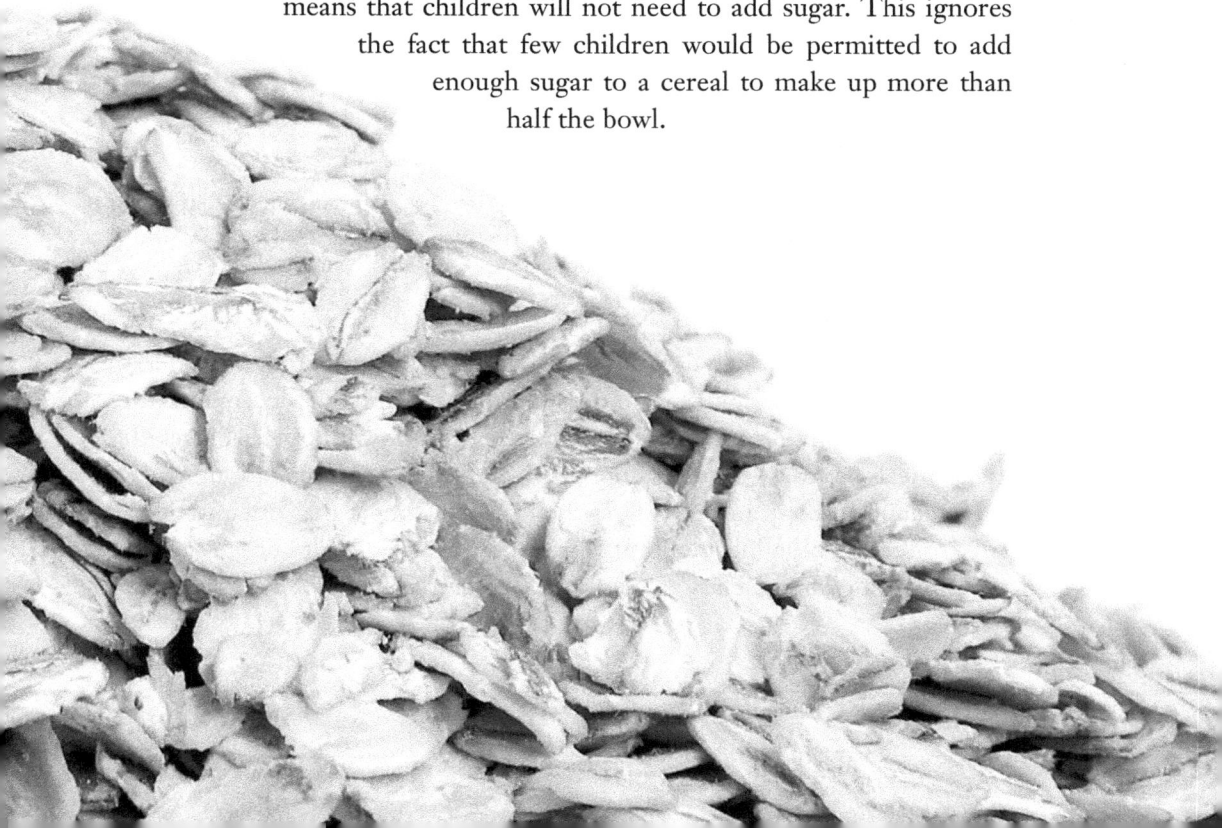

How to judge a breakfast cereal

- *Serving size*. This is determined by the manufacturer and may be quite different from what you would normally eat – and vary between basically similar products. Check the various serving sizes listed. It is often easiest to make comparisons between products from the 'per 100 g' column.
- *Wholegrain*. Look for this word on the package and in the ingredient list. Refined cereals have much less value.
- *Dietary fibre*. Look for at least 10 g fibre per 100 g.
- *Sugar*. If the cereal contains dried fruit, this may be contributing much of the sugar content. If no dried fruit is present, choose products with the lowest sugar content. In general, 100 g of a good value cereal should have less than 10 g sugar (apart from that contributed by dried fruit).
- *Sodium*. There is no technical reason for salt being added to breakfast cereals. Some ingredients will contain small amounts of naturally occurring sodium, but the sodium content should be as low as possible, preferably less than 120 mg/100 g.
- *Fat*. Seeds, nuts and oats contain healthy unsaturated fats. This is not a problem.
- *Saturated fat*. Check the nutrition information panel because higher levels of saturated fat mean that fats – which may include trans fat – have been added. Levels above 1.5 g saturated fat per 100 g are undesirable and usually only occur in 'toasted' mueslis and baked, broken-cluster type cereals. Most of these products are also high in added sugar. Choose a quality muesli instead. Or make your own from my recipe.
- *Vitamins*. Most breakfast cereals add vitamins B1, B2 and B3. These are almost never low in the diet and while none are harmful in excess, adding them to a high-sugar cereal does not turn it into a healthy choice.
- *Other additives*. Cereals with added colourings or other numbered additives are almost always also high in sugar. Give them a miss.

Symbols on packets

Manufacturers can buy various symbols for products that fit the criteria set by particular sponsoring organisations. Australia's Glycemic Index Foundation sells a G for products that meet its low GI criteria. Over 40 cereals sport a red tick of approval from the Heart Foundation, which manufacturers can only buy if their products meet that organisation's criteria. These include limits for saturated fat and salt and a requirement for some dietary fibre, but manufacturers can still buy the tick if their products contain 30 per cent or more of added sugar. Check the ingredients on these products. Some expensive rolled oats with the tick have added inulin (a form of dietary fibre) but also dilute the goodness of the oats with 20 per cent wheat starch.

DID YOU KNOW?

- Cornflakes have more salt than potato crisps.
- Wheatgerm is packed with naturally occurring nutrients, providing a good source of protein, dietary fibre, essential fatty acids, zinc, iron, potassium, magnesium, vitamin E, and the B vitamins thiamin (B1), niacin (B3), folate, vitamin B6, pantothenic acid and biotin.
- Oats are oats. Boxed products may be five times the price of house brand oats, but the main difference is that the more expensive products have been checked to ensure that you don't get the odd bit of husk.
- Quick-cooking oats are merely oats that have been sliced more finely so they will cook faster. This reduces the time they take to be digested, so regular oats may keep you feeling full longer.
- To reduce the time for cooking regular rolled oats, place the oats in a saucepan, add milk or water and leave in the fridge overnight. Next morning, add hot water, bring to the boil and your porridge is ready.
- Wheat biscuit cereals are usually the cheapest processed cereal and also among the most nutritious, being made from whole grain, with less than 3 per cent sugar and a low salt content.

Butter or margarine
– which and why?

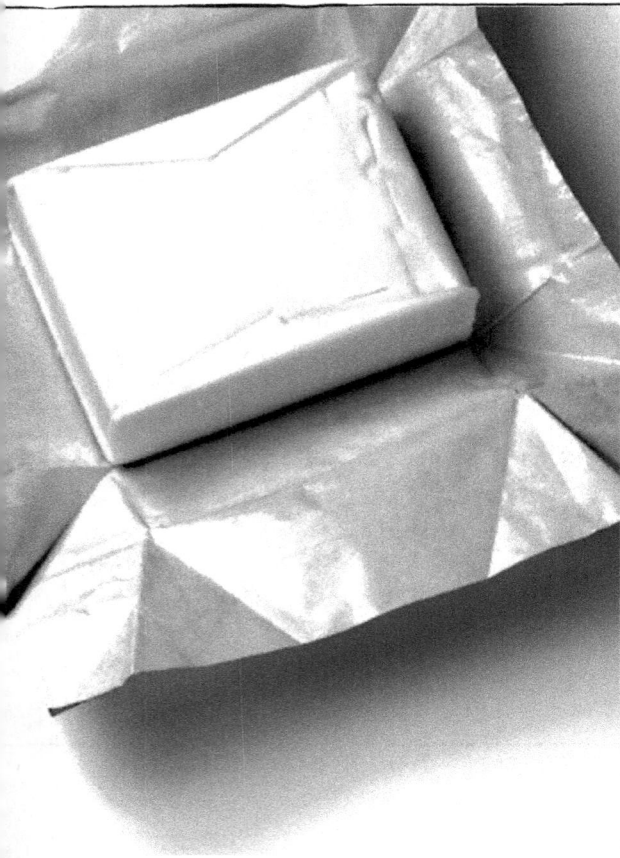

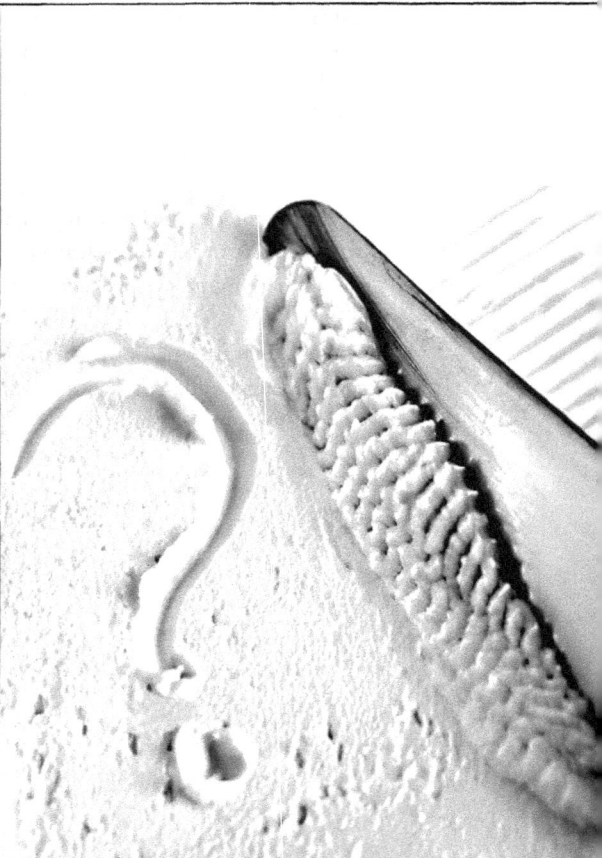

WHENEVER I HAVE WRITTEN on this topic over the years, I have been damned by the sellers of both products. The truth is that neither product is all good or all bad and, as with most fatty products, moderation is the key. I must admit, however, that I do not and will not eat margarine, and even though I love the taste of butter I cannot in conscience describe it as a healthy food.

Butter

Historians believe that butter was probably made accidentally, at least as far back as 3500 BC, when nomadic tribes carried milk in leather bags during their long journeys.

These days, butter is churned from cream separated from milk. It is easy to make and can be made in the home kitchen by beating cream until water separates from the curd. Once the curds are drained and the water is squeezed out, you have butter which can be consumed as it is or salted for longer keeping.

Among spreads, butter wins easily for taste. As children, we ate our vegetables, partly because we were told to do so, but also because a piece of butter on top made the vegetables taste appealing. Butter is also the product of choice for baking as its flavour comes through in pastries, cakes and biscuits. Few professional chefs will use a shortening other than butter – mainly because butter tastes so much better than any other form of shortening.

Butter also scores well for being a more natural product with no need for colourings, preservatives or other additives. Indeed, the only permitted additive to Australian butter is salt. Unsalted butter is also widely available and is the preferred spread in most European countries, as well as being favoured by chefs and for many applications in baking. Australian butter is yellow because our cows live outside eating green grass containing a high quantity of natural yellow-coloured pigments. Colouring is not a permitted additive in Australian butter. In parts of Europe where cows are kept indoors in winter and fed dried material, which has very little of the natural pigments, butter is paler in colour. American cows are usually grain-fed and also produce pale butter.

Butter is approximately 80 per cent fat, of which about two thirds is in the form of saturated fatty acids. Its only real nutritional contribution comes from its high content of pre-formed vitamin A (also called retinol). Butter contains some vitamin E and small quantities of iodine and vitamin D. Butter also contains some ready-made cholesterol, but this is of little consequence since most excess cholesterol in the body comes from the body's own over-production. The amount of cholesterol in a 10 g pat of butter is 14 mg. For comparison, a piece of lean grilled steak contains about 130 mg. The body tends to make too much cholesterol when the diet is high in saturated fat and it is this component of butter that is of potential concern.

Margarine

Emperor Louis Napoleon III is credited as the father of the margarine industry; he offered a reward to anyone who could make a butter substitute that could be used by the armed forces and the poor. The first margarine was made for him in 1869 and patented in 1873; its recipe included animal fats churned with milk and salt for flavour. Initially legislators did not permit margarine to be coloured and its rather unattractive appearance curtailed its use. Some hard margarines are still made from animal fats but most table margarines are now made from processed vegetable oils.

The processing starts by de-gumming the oils – usually cottonseed, sunflower, canola or corn. The oils are then treated with a strong alkali such as caustic soda to remove free fatty acids that would cause rancidity, washed with hot water and dried before being bleached using a mixture of bleaching earth and charcoal. The earth and charcoal are then filtered out. The next step is to deodorise the oil, usually by heating it and blowing steam through it. The oil is now colourless, odourless and tasteless. Various techniques are then used to harden some of it to create a spreadable consistency. Partial hydrogenation is used in some countries but this produces trans fat and is no longer used in Australia. Other methods use processes known as 'fractionation' or 'rearrangement' to convert just enough of the oil's unsaturated fat into saturated fat to produce a spread. Following the addition of whey, water, emulsifiers, salt, colouring and vitamins A and D, the product is then pasteurised and packaged.

NUTRIENTS

Legislation once deemed that margarine should contain 80 per cent fat, just like butter. These days, most margarines contain 70 per cent fat and must be labelled as 'spreads' rather than margarines. Some reduced-fat spreads have 50 per cent fat and extra water, often with milk powder and more emulsifiers added. Vitamins A, E and D are added, with some products having a slightly greater content of vitamin E than butter, but less vitamin A. The fat content in margarines and spreads varies but is usually 20–25 per cent saturated fat, with monounsaturated fats predominating if the product is made from canola and olive oils, and polyunsaturated fats the major type if the spread is made from corn, sunflower, safflower or soy oil. Products with olive oil in their name usually contain at least 50 per cent canola oil. Apart from the monounsaturated fat, they do not retain the beneficial components found in extra virgin olive oil.

PLANT STEROL-ENRICHED SPREADS

A relatively new range of spreads (and other products) contain added compounds called phytosterols (or plant sterols). Phytosterols prevent cholesterol being absorbed from the small intestine into the bloodstream, although they do not get rid of cholesterol deposits already in the arteries. The phytosterol currently permitted in Australia, sitosterol, is extracted from soy

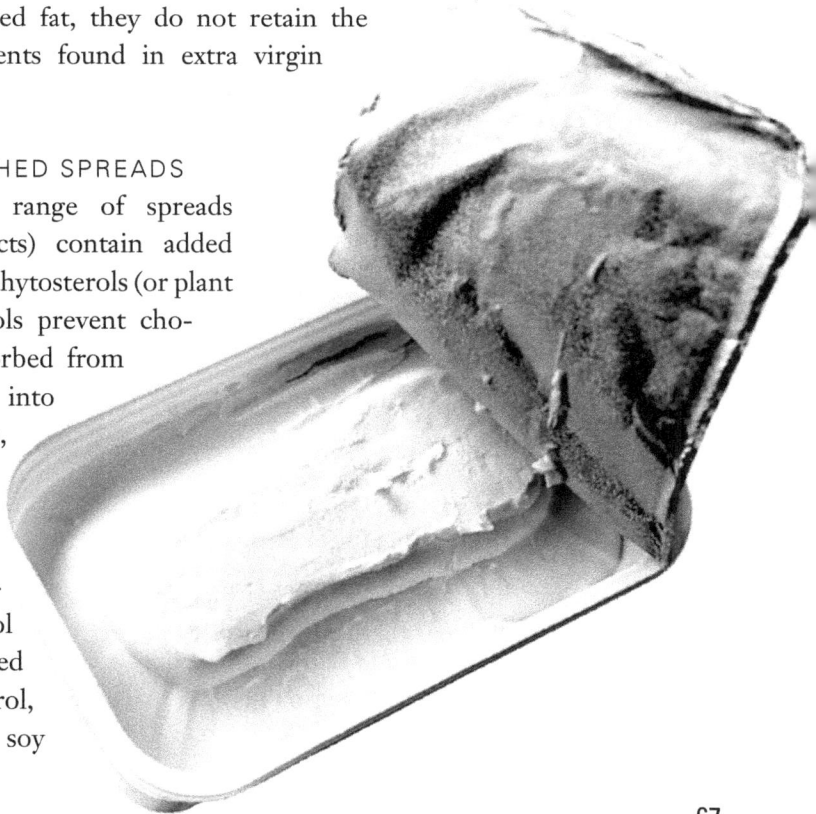

67

beans. In some countries sitostanol, another product with similar action, is extracted from wood pulp. These spreads are labelled as 'reducing cholesterol absorption' because it is illegal to claim that a food will reduce blood cholesterol.

Short-term studies show that these phytosterols can reduce cholesterol levels by 8–10 per cent. Other studies show, however, that phytosterols also reduce the absorption of valuable food components, especially the carotenoids found in fruits and vegetables. Most studies have only checked the effects on the carotenoids alpha and beta carotene and lycopene, and a form of vitamin E called alpha tocopherol. In all cases, the levels of these protective compounds are reduced when products with added plant sterols are included in the diet. CSIRO scientists found that the adverse effects on carotenoids could be overcome if those consuming these spreads also ate an extra serving of fruit and vegetables each day. This seems like cold comfort when few people eat even the recommended quantities of fruit and vegetables.

Spreads containing plant sterols cost up to four times as much as other spreads and the extraction of the plant sterol from soy beans is an expensive and environmentally wasteful process. Five hectares of soy beans are needed to produce 1 kilogram of plant sterols and while the rest of the soy bean can be used for animal fodder, this is a poor use of land, fertiliser and water.

Plant sterol spreads are not a magic bullet, they do not attack the underlying cause of high cholesterol (which is consumption of too many foods high in saturated fat), they lead to the loss of potentially valuable compounds which may have anti-cancer properties, and they are expensive. And, of course, they still taste like margarine.

The take-home message

Being biased against margarine, and wary of the high saturated fat content of butter, my solution is to use olive oil for cooking and on vegetables and salads, and use only small amounts of butter. A freshly made sandwich doesn't need any kind of 'yellow grease'.

Chocolate

– is it good for us or just heavenly?

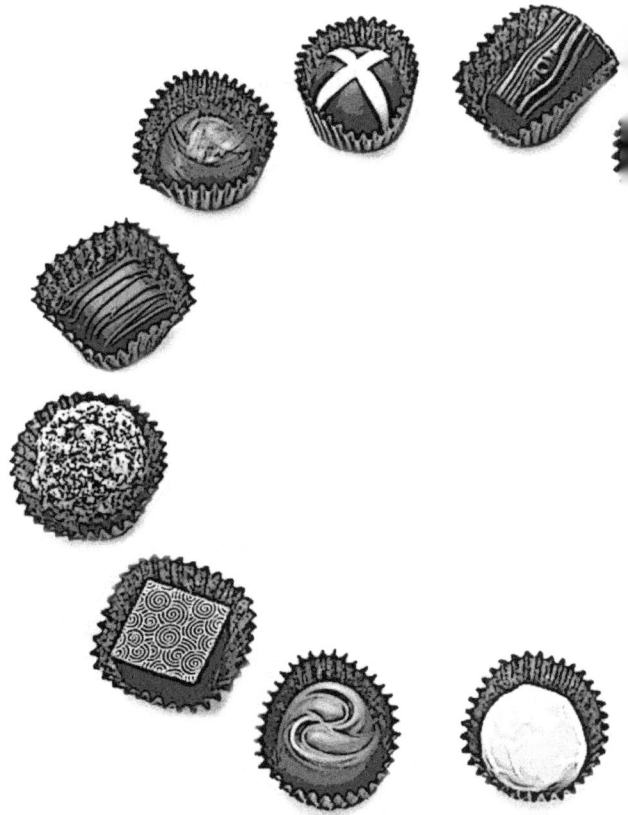

ABOUT 4000 YEARS AGO, when Mayan civilisations in South America 'discovered' chocolate, they deemed it 'divine' – the food of the gods. Modern-day chocoholics agree. Chocolate packs fats, sugar, some nutrients and plenty of kilojoules into a small package, making it an important survival food in times of scarcity. For most other people, however, a high load of kilojoules, fat and sugar can be a recipe for nutritional disaster. Countering that, chocolate is now being hailed as a health food!

The story of chocolate

Children would like chocolate to grow on trees – and it does! Cacao trees grow mainly in West Africa and Brazil and also in parts of New Guinea, although you can't go and pick yourself a chocolate. The fruit of the chocolate tree comes in pods. When the pods ripen, they burst open to release 20 to 40 beans, which are laid out to dry, roasted, and ground to a powder which is intensely bitter.

The Mayans roasted the cacao beans and pounded them to a powder, mixed it with chilli and corn and allowed the mixture to ferment. The Aztecs, who believed chocolate had great restorative powers, also made a drink from the roasted ground beans, adding pepper, vanilla and water. The Spanish explorer Hernando Cortez first tasted this bitter-sweet drink at the court of Montezuma in Mexico in 1519; he

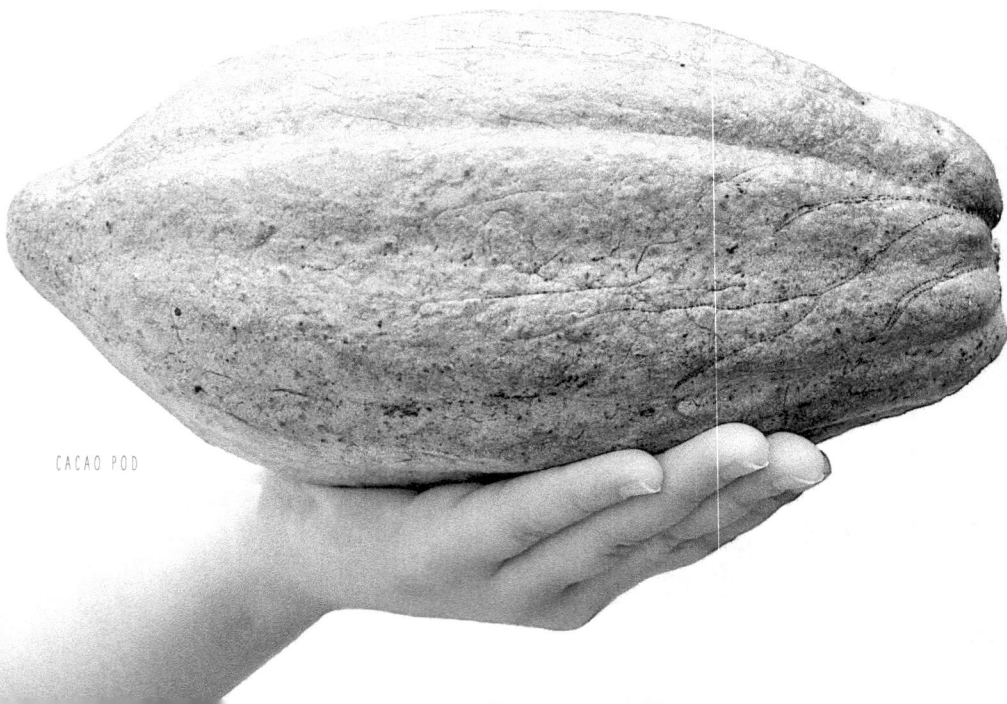

CACAO POD

took chocolate back to Spain where it was greatly revered. During the sixteenth century in Europe the drink was used to treat emaciated patients or as a vehicle to counteract the unpleasant taste of various medicinal herbs. Gradually chocolate became popular throughout Europe. When Princess Anne of Austria married King Louis XIII in the seventeenth century she introduced chocolate to the French, who added sugar, spices and almonds or hazelnuts, still using it as a drink. The first chocolate house opened in London in 1657 and the popularity of the sweet drink spread rapidly.

In 1828 the Dutchman Johannes van Houten built a machine to separate the cocoa butter from the cocoa beans, making a powder that could easily be mixed with sugar for chocolate drinks. This paved the way for the solid chocolate bars that are now the major form in which chocolate is consumed. The first chocolate bars were made in England in 1847. In 1875 the first milk chocolate was made in Switzerland; milk chocolate has become the most popular type of chocolate in the world.

These days, the cocoa butter and powder are blended with sugar, with the best quality chocolate having a higher percentage of the cocoa butter and powder. Cheaper chocolates have less of the real ingredients and more added fats plus emulsifiers and other additives. Milk chocolate has milk powder or condensed milk added.

Why we love it

Humans are born with a love of sweet foods. Most people also love anything with a warm creamy mouth-feel, so chocolate's sensory properties almost certainly contribute to its seductive qualities. Chocolate also contains some potentially addictive substances, including a stimulant called theobromine, tyramine (an amino acid), phenylethylamine (related to amphetamine) and anadamide (related to compounds found in cannabis). It's tempting to assume that these compounds are responsible for chocolate 'addiction', but their quantities are too small to cause a true addiction. For those seeking a 'hit', dark chocolate has more theobromine than milk chocolate.

One placebo-controlled British study has reported that the quantity of theobromine and caffeine in a 50 g bar of chocolate (milk or dark) can improve reaction times, processing of visual information and what the researchers called 'energy arousal'. White chocolate (which does not contain these compounds) was no more effective than water. While the researchers thought it likely that the two compounds contributed to chocolate's popularity, its taste and sensory properties were likely to be even greater reasons for its popularity.

Chocolate also contains a small amount of caffeine, but if you're after stimulation, you'll do much better with a coffee – since 100 g of chocolate has ōnly as much caffeine as a cup of pathetically weak tea.

Chocolate and your health

ANTIOXIDANTS

The sellers of chocolate have funded and publicised a number of studies that consistently show chocolate is rich in antioxidants. The research may be valid, but most studies used cocoa extracts and any benefits apply mainly to expensive bitter chocolate, not the average milk chocolate bar. At present the way cocoa is processed for use in regular chocolate removes about 90 per cent of the antioxidant compounds. The companies funding these studies are keen to isolate the antioxidant components of the cocoa bean so they can be added in concentrated form to the more popular sweet chocolate bars and other chocolate confectionery products. Until that occurs, if you want the antioxidants in chocolate, you need to go for the imported bitter variety. The potency of the antioxidants in dark chocolate also needs further study. If you are after antioxidants, the top sources include fruits, vegetables, whole grains and extra virgin olive oil.

BLOOD PRESSURE

An analysis of 13 studies on the effects of chocolate on blood pressure found that dark chocolate is superior to a placebo (usually white chocolate) in reducing blood pressure, although the effect is slight and occurs only in those with slightly raised pressure. The effective quantity is small too – one small square a day. Researchers also caution that chocolate should be used in place of, not in addition to, other high-kilojoule foods and snacks.

Some claim it is the flavanol antioxidants, others believe it is the theobromine in chocolate, that stimulate the body to produce nitric oxide – which relaxes blood vessels, thus allowing an increased flow of blood to the heart, brain and other body organs. For the record, nuts have a much greater ability to increase production of nitric oxide within the body – chocolate-coated almonds, anyone?

CHOLESTEROL

The chocolate industry often claims that a particular saturated fat in chocolate called stearic acid won't raise cholesterol. This is correct – in part. Chocolate is also a rich source of another saturated fat, called palmitic acid, which many studies show can increase blood cholesterol. Most chocolate contains almost as much of the undesirable palmitic acid as the less problematic stearic acid. It would be foolish to think chocolate can control your cholesterol.

DENTAL DECAY

Japanese research claims chocolate protects teeth from decay. Little publicity is given to the fact that these studies showed that it was the *husk* of the cocoa bean, which is discarded in making chocolate, that was the source of the protective compound that might stop the formation of plaque. (Bacteria in plaque convert food carbohydrates to acids, which then erode the enamel on teeth to cause cavities.) The studies reported a reduction in dental decay in rats fed the cocoa bean husk and suggested that the active compound from the husk might be suitable as an additive to toothpaste.

On the other hand, compared with most sugary confectionery, chocolate *is* less likely to cause dental decay, mainly because its fat content provides a slight buffer against sugar's damaging effects.

Is it fattening?

Whether any food is fattening depends on how much of it you eat. Chocolate is one of the most concentrated sources of kilojoules available, so go easy on the quantity. A 100 g bar of milk or dark chocolate contains approximately 28 g of fat (mostly saturated fat) and a good third of daily energy requirements at 2170 kJ.

Energy food?

Many people crave chocolate when they feel in need of an energy boost, and chocolate's high kilojoule content certainly gives it the right to be called an 'energy food'. But if you want a quick burst of energy, forget chocolate. Its high fat content means it takes time to be digested and release its sugar into the bloodstream. The 'boost' that many people claim after eating chocolate is a psychological one and it probably stems largely from the pleasure of its sweet creaminess in the mouth. For a quick burst of energy, a banana is a better bet.

Which chocolate?

DARK

Dark chocolate – especially the bitter, expensive brands – contains the highest level of antioxidants. Dark chocolate is also a good source of magnesium, iron and zinc.

MILK

Milk chocolate, with its added milk powder, scores points for calcium, with five times the quantity found in dark chocolate.

WHITE

White chocolate is made of deodorised cocoa butter with added milk and sugar. It may have a slight chocolate flavour from the cocoa butter but it's not strictly chocolate as it does not contain the thick chocolate 'liquor' made after fermenting, roasting and grinding the cacao bean. The milk content does provide some calcium, but its added fats are saturated.

COOKING

Compounded cooking chocolate is made from solid vegetable fats, sugar and cocoa. Its fats are more likely to raise blood cholesterol than other types of chocolate.

The bottom line

Chocolate is a treat rather than a treatment. Why not enjoy a small portion for its divine taste?

Coffee

– our favourite addiction

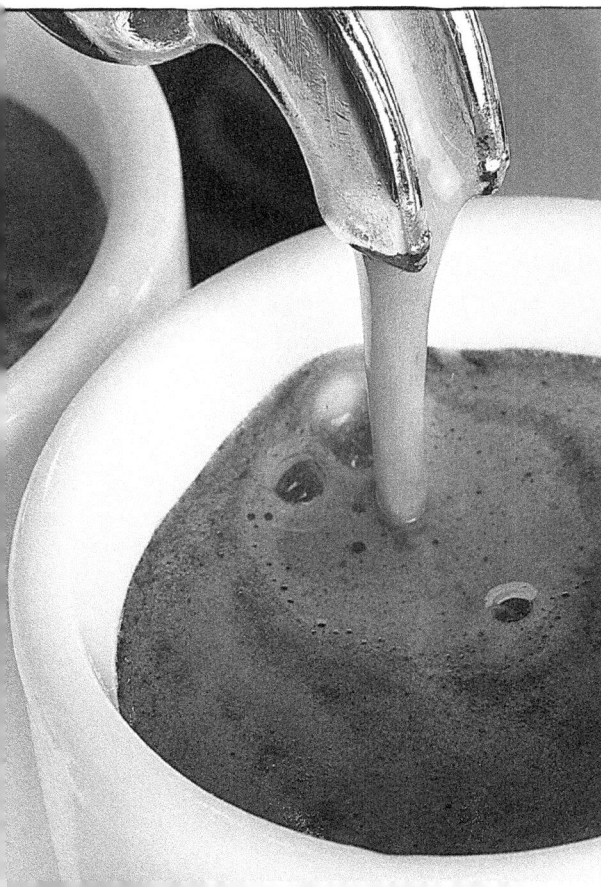

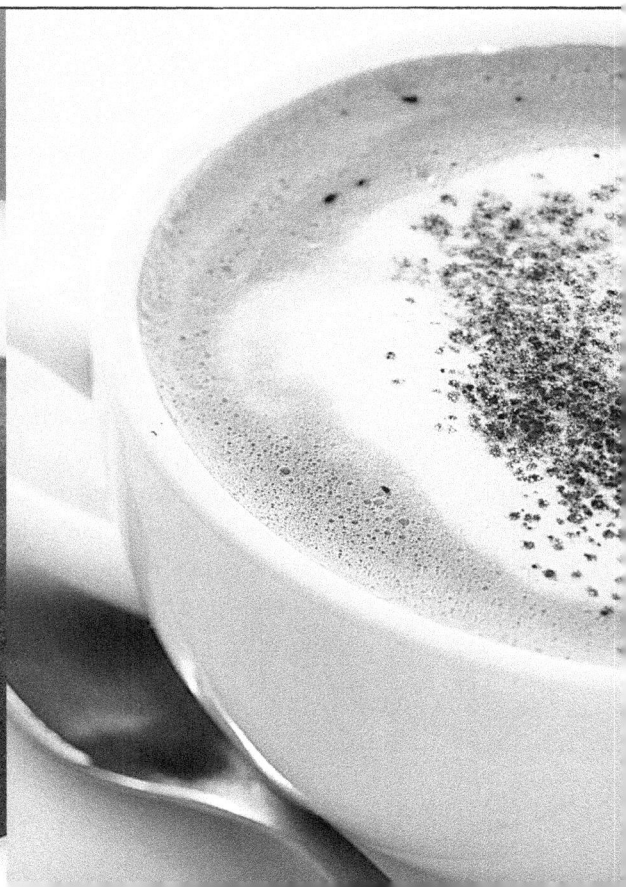

FEW OF US WHO DRINK COFFEE consider ourselves drug addicts – but we should. Its caffeine is addictive in the true sense of the word. And as with any addiction, if we don't get our usual hit we develop symptoms that commonly include headaches, irritability, fatigue and lack of mental alertness. A caffeine hit and we're back feeling fine! Caffeine is the most widely used drug throughout the world. It wakes us up and improves reaction times. The good news is that most people can keep the addiction to reasonable levels where the caffeine is unlikely to do any harm and may have some beneficial effects. However, if you need surgery, note that the 'nil-by-mouth' requirement includes caffeine deprivation – which is the cause of some post-operative headaches.

The caffeine content of coffee depends on the type of coffee bean used, with the more expensive Arabica beans (*Coffea arabica*) having less caffeine than the Robusta type (*Coffea canephora robusta*) used for instant coffee. Drinking coffee may also have other advantages. Apart from the enjoyment it affords, coffee is a good source of antioxidants. It may be addictive, but we can still enjoy coffee – in moderation.

Coffee and health

HEART DISEASE, DIABETES, STROKE, GOUT, DEMENTIA, ASTHMA

A study of almost 60 000 men and women in Finland recently found coffee had no adverse effects on heart disease. When other factors were taken into account, 3–4 cups of coffee a day had a protective effect against heart failure. Studies in Japan and Sweden also show that regular consumption of up to 3 cups of coffee a day reduces the risk of dying from heart disease. Researchers have also shown that a regular intake of 2–4 cups of coffee a day is beneficial for those with diabetes because it increases insulin sensitivity; 2–4 cups of coffee also reduce the risk of stroke and gout. Those who drink coffee in mid-life also have 65 per cent less risk of developing dementia in later life. For asthma sufferers, a cup of coffee can improve airway function for 2–4 hours afterwards.

Coffee contains some polyphenols that function as helpful antioxidants. One, called chlorogenic acid, is metabolised in the intestine to an even more powerful antioxidant called caffeic acid. These acids may be responsible for some of the favourable effects of coffee.

76

BLOOD PRESSURE

Where studies show adverse effects of coffee on blood pressure or other health markers, it is usually because the subjects are not regular coffee drinkers. If you aren't used to coffee, it can increase blood pressure. Some people also find coffee alters their usual heart rhythm, although this depends on the dose. Drinking several cups can have adverse effects on several markers of heart disease, but when coffee is consumed regularly, it appears to have little effect on blood pressure or most other markers of cardiovascular disease.

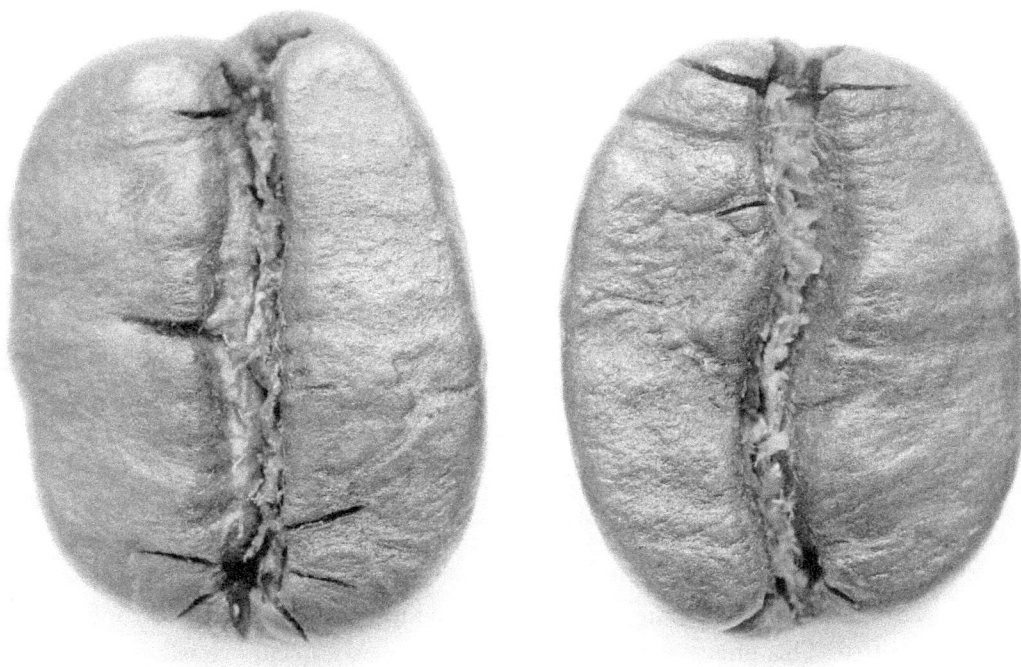

CHOLESTEROL

Controversy continues over whether coffee raises cholesterol, but it's interesting to note where the studies are carried out. Those from the United States usually show little effect of coffee consumption on cholesterol, possibly because the coffee consumed in the United States is weak and usually filtered. European studies are more likely to show adverse effects on blood cholesterol or heart rhythm, especially among heavy coffee drinkers, possibly because European coffee is strong.

77

Coffee contains small amounts of diterpenes, including substances called kahweol and cafestol. Both have the potential to raise cholesterol, but it depends on how the coffee is prepared. Turkish coffee, and coffee that is boiled or made in a plunger pot, have relatively high levels of diterpenes and may have a cholesterol-raising effect. Instant, percolated and filtered coffee contain virtually no cafestol and kahweol and do not appear to raise cholesterol. Espresso has only small quantities and also appears to be safe. If unfiltered, both Arabica and Robusta coffee beans can raise cholesterol, but as Robusta coffee contains very little kahweol, researchers in the Netherlands have deduced that cafestol is the culprit.

WEIGHT LOSS

Don't count on coffee for weight loss. Claims that coffee increases metabolic rate only apply to those who don't normally drink coffee – after a few days, the body gets used to the effect of the coffee and it ceases to make any difference to metabolic rate.

BONE DENSITY

Claims that coffee reduces bone density are only valid for those who drink more than 10 cups a day. Smaller amounts do not have adverse effects, and when coffee is taken as a latte or cappuccino the milk makes a positive contribution to bone health. Almost a third of all milk consumed in Australia is in coffee.

INDIGESTION

Some people get indigestion after drinking coffee, especially strong coffee. This effect is not due to the caffeine as it occurs equally with decaffeinated coffee. The problem may lie with coffee's acidic components. Ovderindulgence in strong coffee can occasionally cause painful oesophageal spasm, which feels like violent heartburn.

Coffee and alcohol

Coffee does not undo the effects of alcohol. A strong coffee after drinking will not assist you to drive and has no ability to hasten the metabolism of alcohol. It is a potentially dangerous myth that someone who

78

has been drinking is fit to drive after a strong coffee. Caffeine may make someone believe they are awake enough to drive, but neither coffee nor any other form of caffeine improves reaction times. The combination of alcohol with caffeine from energy drinks is particularly hazardous (see pages 89–90).

Does it keep you awake?

Many people claim that coffee does not keep them awake whereas others find that coffee after dinner or even drunk late afternoon means a sleepless night. Both may be correct and somewhat ironically, those who consume the least coffee tend to be most strongly affected if they have an evening cup.

How much coffee?

Consumption of 2–3 cups of coffee a day appears safe for most people. Those who suffer from insomnia should avoid coffee after about 4 pm.

Coffee for children

The dose of caffeine in a cup of coffee or tea is proportionately much larger for a child than an adult, and can have adverse effects, particularly in terms of hyperactivity. Some cases of hyperactivity disappear when the child stops consuming caffeine. Children who are permitted to drink coffee or tea also tend to drink less milk. Teenagers may use coffee to stay awake for studying or partying. This is not a good idea as teenagers need adequate sleep.

Coffee and pregnancy

Some studies show that caffeinated beverages reduce fertility in both men and women; others show no effect from moderate intake. Many women find an aversion to coffee is the first sign of pregnancy. This may be nature's warning, as some studies show that spontaneous abortion in the first trimester of pregnancy is more likely in women who consume several cups of coffee a day. Caffeine metabolism is also much slower during pregnancy and it does cross the placenta. Whether babies

79

become addicted to caffeine before birth is controversial. However, it appears that a high caffeine intake while breastfeeding leads to restless babies who don't sleep well. As a result, it is wise for women to restrict their coffee intake during pregnancy and while breastfeeding: 1–2 cups a day is probably safe.

Decaffeinated coffee?

For those who are sensitive to caffeine or wish to reduce their intake, decaffeinated coffee is helpful. Coffee is decaffeinated by several methods:

- using a chemical solvent (usually trichlorethylene)
- using steam
- soaking green beans in water, which allows the caffeine to migrate to the outer surface of the bean, which is then removed by abrasion.

COMPARE THE CAFFEINE

Coffee, instant, average mug	60–90 mg
Coffee, espresso or brewed, average cup	80–120 mg
Tea, strong, average cup	50–60 mg
Tea, weak, average cup	20–30 mg
Cola drinks, 370 mL	30–35 mg
Chocolate, 100 g	10–30 mg
Chocolate milk, 250 mL	10–20 mg
Energy drinks, 375 mL	50–500 mg

Eggs
– good, bad, and good again

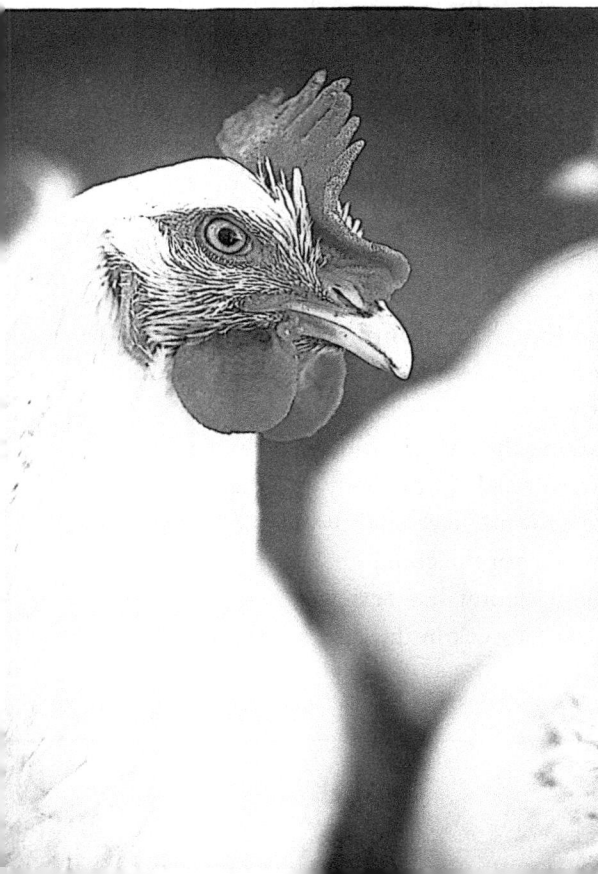

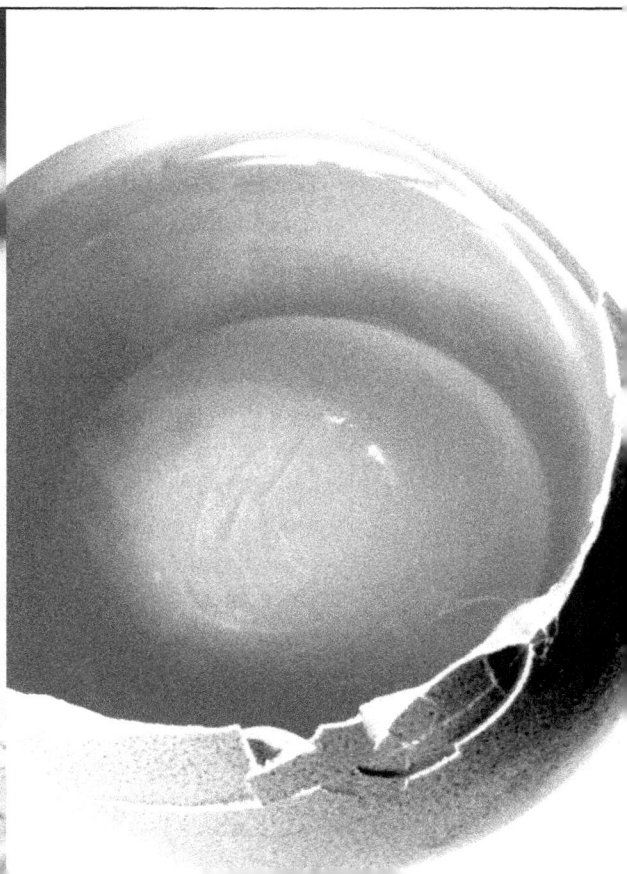

WHEN I WAS A CHILD, EGGS were a staple part of weekday breakfasts, almost always served with bacon and often with the addition of a chop, sausage or baked beans. Hard-working men and hungry teenagers often got eggs with the lot! On weekends, we were allowed to skip the cooked breakfast and have just cereal and toast. At the time, average consumption of eggs was 255 a year, or five a week. Jump forward a few years to the time when most women started working outside the home and the cooked breakfast disappeared – at least during the week. Eggs still made an occasional appearance on Sunday mornings.

Eggs and cholesterol

The demise of the cooked breakfast coincided with advice from the Heart Foundation to restrict eggs to no more than two a week. Egg consumption halved. So why did the Heart Foundation (and others) take such a savage swipe at eggs in the late 1960s? At that time, heart attacks were common in men in their forties, fifties and sixties, especially if they were smokers, as many more were in those days. There was also a strong correlation between heart attacks and blood levels of cholesterol. Researchers also showed that blood cholesterol rose with a higher intake of saturated fat. When people ate saturated fat, the body made more of this waxy cholesterol and some of it clogged the arteries.

The 'big breakfast' was high in saturated fat, mainly from the fat on bacon and chops and in sausages. Eggs are not particularly high in saturated fat, although they contain some. Like all animal foods, however, eggs contain some ready-made cholesterol. Researchers were aware that saturated fat (present in foods in gram quantities) was much more at fault than ready-made cholesterol (present in milligram quantities), but 'experts' considered that it was hard enough to get people to pronounce 'cholesterol' without adding the complication that there might be a difference between cholesterol made in the body and that present in foods. So because eggs (and prawns) have slightly higher levels of ready-made cholesterol, both foods got the chop!

More recently, the Heart Foundation has reviewed the evidence and decided that including six eggs a week in the diet is not associated with coronary heart disease. They therefore allow eggs to carry their familiar tick.

The bottom line

Some of us never subscribed to the idea that eggs were a problem food. The big daily breakfast fry-up was a problem because of its high saturated fat content, but the poor egg did not deserve to be tarred with that brush. Two eggs have less saturated fat than the average amount of 'unsaturated' margarine spread on the breakfast toast.

How nutritious are eggs?

Nature has designed eggs to support a growing chicken. They are a good source of high quality protein, iron, zinc, selenium, iodine and a range of vitamins including A, E and six of the eight vitamins of the B complex (riboflavin, niacin, biotin, folate, pantothenic acid and B12). Egg yolks are also rich in two carotenoid pigments, lutein and zeaxanthin, both important for the health of the retina in the eye. Spinach and other green vegetables also supply these pigments but their absorption is greater from eggs. An average-sized egg has about 6 g of fat, with only 2 g as saturated fat and the rest as healthy unsaturated fat. Cholesterol content is about 250 mg per egg.

Almost everyone needs a quick meal at times. You need only minutes to make a spinach or mushroom omelette and, compared with a fast food alternative, the omelette will have more valuable nutrients and a fraction of the fat.

Which egg?

FREE-RANGE

Free-range hens have protection from the elements but can also roam outside, scratch about in dirt to forage for food or dust bathe, flap their wings, perch and socialise.

BARN LAID

Barn laid eggs are from animals that can move freely around large sheds.

CAGE

Cage eggs come from hens kept in cages with very little room to move (each hens usually has an area about the size of an A4 piece of paper).

In Australia, the RSPCA continues to push for a ban on caged hens and also cites the cruelty of de-beaking hens, which is practised in all three egg-production systems. (De-beaking involves removing a third of the beak to prevent the hen pecking and wounding other hens.) The government is deaf to the RSPCA's pleas, but some supermarkets are phasing out sales of eggs from caged hens. In Sweden, eggs from battery (caged) hens have been banned since 2004. The UK will ban caged hens from January 2012 and most countries across the European Union are moving to follow suit. As some free range hens are still de-beaked, check the source of your eggs carefully.

ORGANIC

Organic eggs come from free-range hens whose feed is organically grown and guaranteed free of genetically modified corn or soy.

No research confirms any nutritional advantages of organic or free range eggs over other eggs, except that eggs from hens that eat fresh greens have deeper coloured yolks with higher levels of some valuable carotenoid pigments.

OMEGA 3-ENRICHED

When hens are fed a supplement of canola or linseed (also called flax-seed) oil, their eggs contain an omega 3 fat called alpha linolenic acid (ALA) which comes from canola or linseeds. Eggs from hens given a fish oil supplement contain omega 3 fats known as EPA and DHA. All types of omega 3s are valuable for health (see page 155). Most omega 3-enriched eggs contain about 90 mg omega 3s per egg. For comparison, 100 g of fish contains 100–600 mg.

The take-home message

The choice of eggs is largely a matter of caring about the way food is produced. As someone who keeps a few happy chooks that can scratch and dig to their heart's content, I refuse to buy eggs from caged hens.

1

Store eggs
in their carton
in the fridge.

2

Eggs age more
in one day at
room temperature
than they do in a
week in the
fridge.

KEEPING
EGGS
FRESH

3

Discard
cracked eggs as
harmful bacteria
can enter through
the cracks.

4

Don't serve raw
eggs to children
under two, pregnant
women or frail
aged people.

Raw eggs
can contain bacteria
that cause serious
health problems for
these groups.

Energy drinks
_– who needs them?

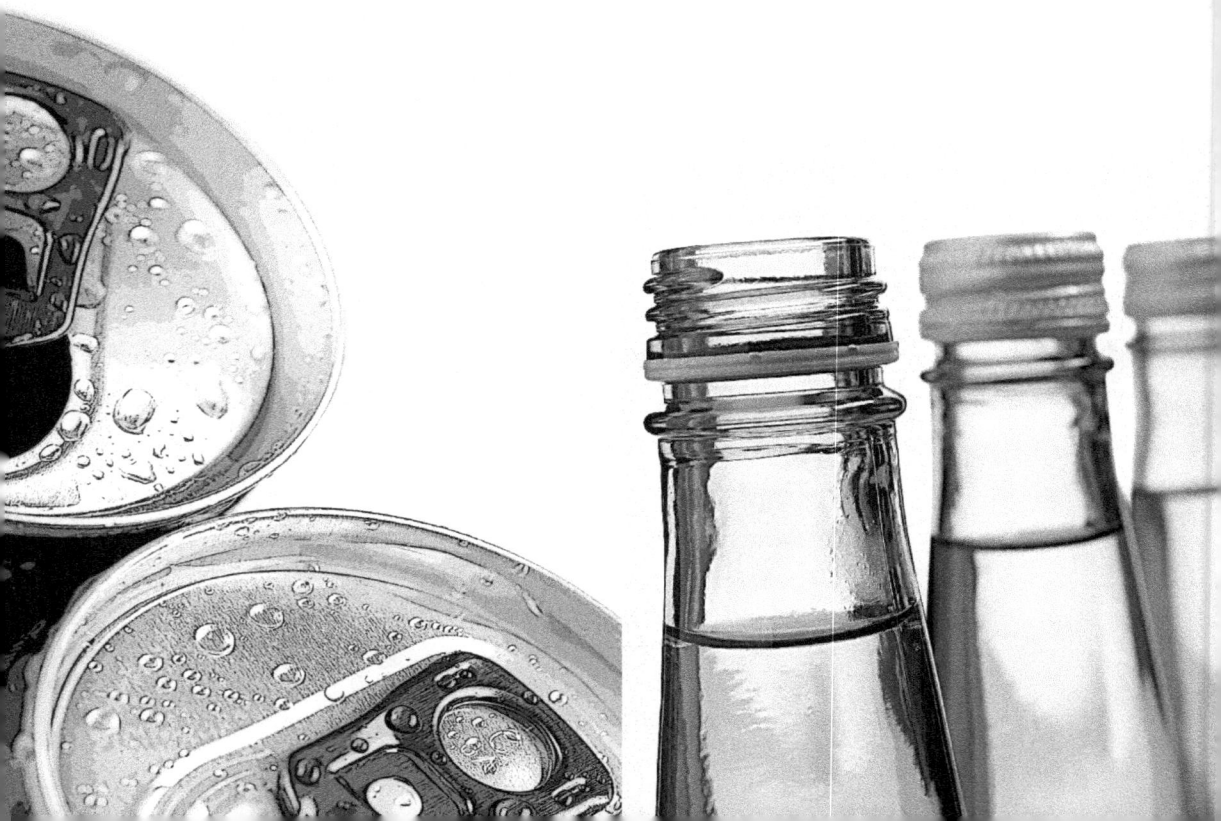

FUELLED BY AGGRESSIVE MARKETING, there is a growing market for adding stimulants to sugared water and selling the mix as an 'energy' drink. It's not all beer and skittles for the marketers, many of whom also sell regular soft drinks. Many of the hundreds of brands of energy drinks launched in Australia over the last 10 years or so have sunk without trace. The ones that have made it aim their marketing thrust at 'red-blooded' young men, and associate the drinks with life in the fast lane, tough sports and implied aggression. The marketing hype implies the drinks will improve stamina and endurance and products are given names that include terms such as jolt, venom, impulse, devil, buzz, hero, jugular, blast, power, sex, wicked, wild or bull. One brand even claims to 'deliver a jolt of energy in new killer packaging'. Before people in emergency departments start hyperventilating, the 'killer packaging' is actually a resealable, recyclable aluminium bottle.

Who buys them?

The claims made for energy drinks have made them popular in gyms and with body builders. Not surprisingly, claims that the products act as a pick-me-up make them popular with students, and claims of better athletic performance make them attractive to teenagers and children. One survey in Sydney found that 27 per cent of eight to 12-year-old children were consuming energy drinks, with some taking up to five cans for 'energy' before sporting events. Other studies also find that about half of 11 to 18-year-olds used energy drinks, mainly as an energy boost.

Energy drinks also appeal to tired, time-poor adults looking for a 'lift'. Truck drivers use them to ward off fatigue. Some people mistakenly think they will undo the effects of alcohol – while some products actually include alcohol.

A few companies have tried to expand the market for energy drinks to women, adding extracts of various herbs, noni fruit or 'magic' berries such as açai or goji to give them a more natural image. But even the high sugar content can't mask the bitterness of the wonder berries and repeat purchases have been disappointing for the promoters. Marketing gurus continue to believe, however, that if they get the formula, taste and marketing right, the sky is the limit for makers of energy drinks.

The ingredients and the facts

- Sugar provides the 'energy' – about 13 teaspoons in a 500 mL can.
- Caffeine is added to give the 'kick' and prevent fatigue. The quantity varies from 50 mg to over 500 mg per can in some imported drinks (a typical cup of coffee has about 80 mg; tea has about 40 mg).
- Guarana, an extract from a South American plant, adds more caffeine, with 1 g of guarana containing caffeine equivalent to a cup of coffee.
- Taurine, an amino acid, is presumably added to provide a reference to the strength of the legendary Taurus (the bull). It is an essential amino acid for cats which, unlike humans (and bulls), are unable to make it within the body.
- Glucuronolactone is a compound normally produced when carbohydrates are broken down within the body.
- B vitamins are included in some products, with no explanation for their presence.
- Herbal ingredients may be listed as ginkgo or ginseng or as 'mystery' ingredients that are claimed to enhance sex urge, vitality, stamina and performance.

DO THESE INGREDIENTS 'WORK'?

For the overweight, the 'energy' (or kilojoules) from the high sugar content is likely to end up as body fat. The drinks are also acidic and promote erosion of the enamel on teeth.

The quantity of caffeine in energy drinks varies. Many brands contain as much caffeine in one can as you would expect from a strong coffee – that is, about twice as much as the equivalent volume of cola. Some of these products, however, have as much caffeine as you would find in 4 or 5 cups of coffee. That's enough to cause nausea or disturbances in heart rhythm in many people, especially teenagers.

Taurine is the second most abundant amino acid in the brain. Its addition to energy drinks is supposedly to 'kickstart metabolism', although there is no evidence to support this notion. Some rodent studies show that a sufficient dose of taurine may produce an anti-anxiety effect in the central nervous system, but other studies (in mice) report that small doses have no stimulant action and no effect on measures of anxiety or depression-like behaviours.

There are no studies on the effects of the glucuronolactone added to energy drinks. Glucuronolactone is a normal metabolite of glucose metabolism and occurs in small quantities in some foods. Wine is the richest dietary source – but energy drinks generally contain up to 500 times the level in wine and any positive or negative effects are unknown. Supplements sold to body-builders claim benefits for performance and energy levels, but again, there is little supporting evidence. The B complex vitamins added to some products are rarely lacking in the Australian diet – and excess quantities are excreted in urine.

Any effect of herbal ingredients added in unknown quantities is likely to be non-existent.

Should energy drinks be banned?

Denmark, Uruguay and Iceland ban the sale of energy drinks and Norway restricts them to pharmacies. Experts in these countries all believe that their safety has not been adequately established. Since the drinks were first produced in Austria in 1997, few tests have been carried out that either support or disprove various manufacturers' claims of 'energy' effects from the combination of ingredients in their products.

Some health authorities are concerned that energy drinks may serve as a gateway to other forms of addictive drugs. Energy drinks with suggestive drug-related names do little to dampen such potential connections. Some studies show a high level of risk-taking behaviour among young people hooked on energy drinks, although there is no suggestion this is due to any ingredient in the drinks.

Combining energy drinks with alcohol is a problem. Contrary to popular belief, energy drinks do not increase the rate at which alcohol is metabolised. Studies show that young men who drink alcohol and then down an energy drink perceive themselves to be sober, report less fatigue, fewer headache symptoms and better coordination. Sadly, an 'alert drunk' is still drunk – and the perception that energy drinks can counteract the effects of alcohol has potentially lethal consequences.

In mid-2008, France lifted its ban on energy drinks, but the government remains concerned about their consumption by children and pregnant women.

Food Standards Australia New Zealand (FSANZ) is reviewing energy drinks. They have set controls over the quantity of stimulants such as caffeine and guarana that can be added, and require labels to note that the products are not suitable for children, pregnant or lactating women

89

or those sensitive to caffeine. The total caffeine content (from both caffeine and guarana) must be provided, along with a general statement that health authorities recommend limiting caffeine intake. No claims can be made about the vitamins or amino acids commonly used in energy drinks, and FSANZ has set maximum quantities for the addition of six B group vitamins, taurine and glucuronolactone. The limit for taurine is 2000 mg per day, and product labels must state that and also the quantity present so that consumers have the information to allow them to stay within this limit.

FSANZ's requirement for the labels on energy drinks to declare an appropriate daily intake may be sensible, but is ignored. One Internet blogger claims: 'Warning High Caffeine Content. OK, we know that's why you're drinking it but our lame legal guys made us warn you not to feed this to kids, up-the-duff women or the weak who just can't tolerate it.' Such sentiments may be generated by energy drinks' marketing.

Research into possible harm mainly centres on the extremely high caffeine content of some of the energy drinks imported into Australia, and on the combination of energy drinks and alcohol. High caffeine levels have led to several deaths in people who did not realise they were sensitive to caffeine. An Adelaide researcher recently found that the combination of caffeine and taurine in energy drinks caused undesirable stickiness in blood platelets in 30 healthy young people. Others in the United States have reported increased heart rates and high blood pressure among healthy young volunteers who consumed two cans of energy drink each day for a week. Australian data shows that young people who combine alcohol with energy drinks both consume more alcohol and increase their risk of getting drunk and engaging in risky alcohol-related behaviours such as drink driving and violence.

The take-home message

Energy drinks are unsuitable for children (as is coffee), teenagers and pregnant women. Adults who are overweight or have cardiovascular problems or a low tolerance to caffeine should avoid them. No one should mix energy drinks with alcohol or assume these products can make up for alcohol's adverse effects.

Fast foods

– time to pause and consider

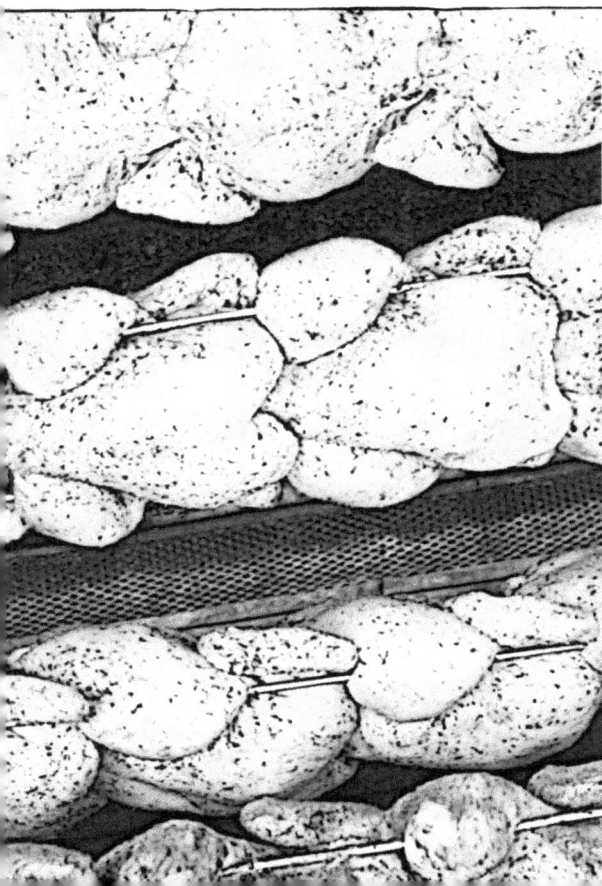

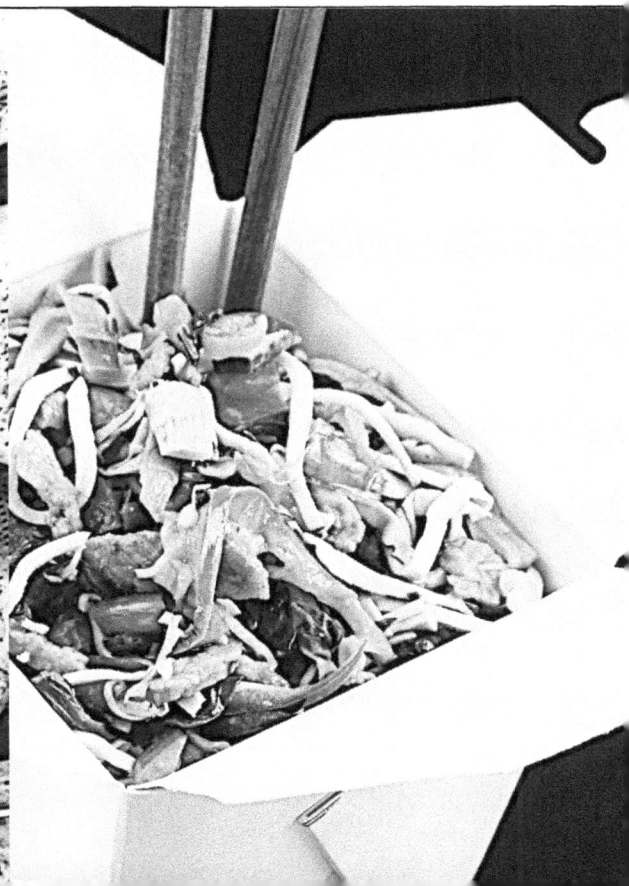

IF THE TERM 'FAST FOODS' were used for those foods which are quickly prepared and served, fresh fruit would be the ultimate fast food. But the 'fast' in this term refers to foods that are available with minimal waiting time and usually can be eaten quickly.

Fast eating comes from the foods being moist (usually achieved with a high fat content) and low in fibre so they need little chewing. Eating quickly interferes with the normal appetite control mechanism, which requires food to stay in the mouth and stomach long enough for gut hormones to send a 'satisfied' signal to the brain – which then sends the message to stop putting food into the mouth. Consider as an example the buns used for fast food burgers. Unlike regular bread, they are high in fat and in particular a fat that melts in the mouth. Combine that with a low-fibre texture and they almost dissolve between the tongue and the roof of the mouth. The moist fatty meat and the 'dissolving' bun can be swallowed with very little chewing. If the contents of a burger are placed in the kind of crusty roll that requires each mouthful to be mixed with saliva and chewed properly before swallowing, the burger will take much longer to eat. And once you have crunched and munched through such a burger, you are likely to feel satisfied and unlikely to eat more. The fast food phenomenon may be good for business, but not for the body.

Are they junk?

Fast foods are often called junk foods, although many contain too many nutrients to really deserve the term. It is their high content of fat, salt and kilojoules, and their almost total lack of vegetables (other than fries) that put them into the junk food category. Some fast food chains have introduced healthier choices, but a recent study found they made up just 2.5 per cent of purchases. The prospect of healthier choices lures more people into the store – but when they get there, they order the same things they normally order. Sales of these products then rise. Having a few healthier options available is just a clever marketing tactic. The attempt by one major chain to sell apples as a healthy option failed – largely, perhaps, because the apples were several times the price of those available in fruit shops.

Are they fattening?

Whether any food is fattening depends on how much of it you eat. Give people easy access to cheap, convenient food that requires little or no chewing and has no flavour that the majority object to, and you have a recipe for overconsumption. Fast foods are high in kilojoules, their presence is ubiquitous and many target children with offers of toys and playgrounds. 'Special meal deals' that offer much more food and drink for not much more money are particularly persuasive. Although many factors contribute to obesity, when these are accounted for, anywhere fast food consumption increases so too does obesity.

Advertising

You have probably never seen an advertisement for a carrot or for most vegetables or fruits, but the fast food sellers advertise relentlessly – their logos are recognised throughout the world. On television, advertisements for fast foods dominate sports programs and programs that children and families watch.

Some fast food companies (now calling themselves 'quick service restaurants') have developed a code for advertising to children in which they pledge to advertise only healthy products. Unfortunately, the code covers only programs shown in very limited hours and doesn't cover times that are much more popular with children (between 6 pm and 9 pm), uses criteria for 'healthy' that nutritionists regard as lax, makes it difficult for parents or the community to complain (since the criteria are not made public) and invokes no punishment for breaches. University studies show that since this initiative was launched, the frequency of advertisements for fast food has stayed unchanged at one an hour per day overall, and at 1.3 advertisements an hour during children's peak viewing times. Without regulation, this is unlikely to change.

In the United States, where the government has required fast food chains to show the calorie content of foods offered, parents have been choosing lower calorie options for their children. (The US uses calories; Australia uses kilojoules for measuring energy content of foods.)

93

Which ones?

BURGERS

In theory, there is nothing nutritionally wrong with a meat patty, salad and bread. In practice, most fast food burgers use fatty, salted meat, a fatty, sweet bun and minimal salad, and added fat and salt in a dollop of sauce and a slice of processed cheese. Checking the kilojoules and fat levels in burgers will become easier when governments require such information to be available at the point of sale.

The interest in health claimed by fast food companies is clearly a sham when they offer a whole day's kilojoules and fat and two days' worth of salt in one big burger. If you care about your health, steer clear in particular of oversized and 'special' burger offers. These 'special offer' products appear to be aimed mainly at young men, and those who succumb frequently are less likely to become old men. Foods like these increase the risk of obesity, high blood pressure, heart attacks and stroke, impotence, diabetes, heart disease and several common cancers.

Smaller burgers or those made by independent outlets are often a better choice. Better quality burgers usually cost more. Making your own with quality bread and lots of salad is by far the best option – and cheaper.

CHICKEN

Fried chicken is high in fat for several reasons: the skin and fat are not trimmed off (and intensively-reared chickens that can't move around much are fatty), the starchy coating soaks up more fat – and the products are deep-fried. The high fat content makes the chicken softer and much easier to eat – and overeat.

Barbecued chicken that rotates on a grill should be, and can be, a healthy product. In most cases, however, as the rotisserie turns fat drips constantly onto the chickens below, resulting in a product that is higher in fat than when a single chicken is cooked this way. The stuffing in barbecued chicken also absorbs fat and adds a high level of salt.

The chicken content in chicken nuggets ranges from 30–60 per cent, with the meat in most brands best described as 'reclaimed'. This means the flesh is mechanically recovered from the scraps left on the bones

94

after breast or thigh fillets are removed. There is nothing wrong with avoiding wastage of this meat, but most manufacturers add starches, gums, fillers, binders, fat (often from chicken skin), sugar, preservatives and water to the chicken mulch before forming the mixture into a shape that can be crumbed and fried. Some varieties contain trans fat and all are high in saturated fat and salt. Straight chicken is a more nutritious choice. Claims that children need nuggets because they are easier to eat than real chicken are absurd. Children have teeth!

CHIPS

Hot chips are the most popular fast food, especially among children. Their fat content varies and depends on the variety of potato, the quality of the oil, how many times the chip is dunked in oil, and the size of the serving. For a given weight, the bigger the chips the lower their surface area and the less fat they will absorb. The fattiest chips are the small, thin, crinkle-cut kind. The least fatty are cut from fresh potatoes and cooked once in quality oil.

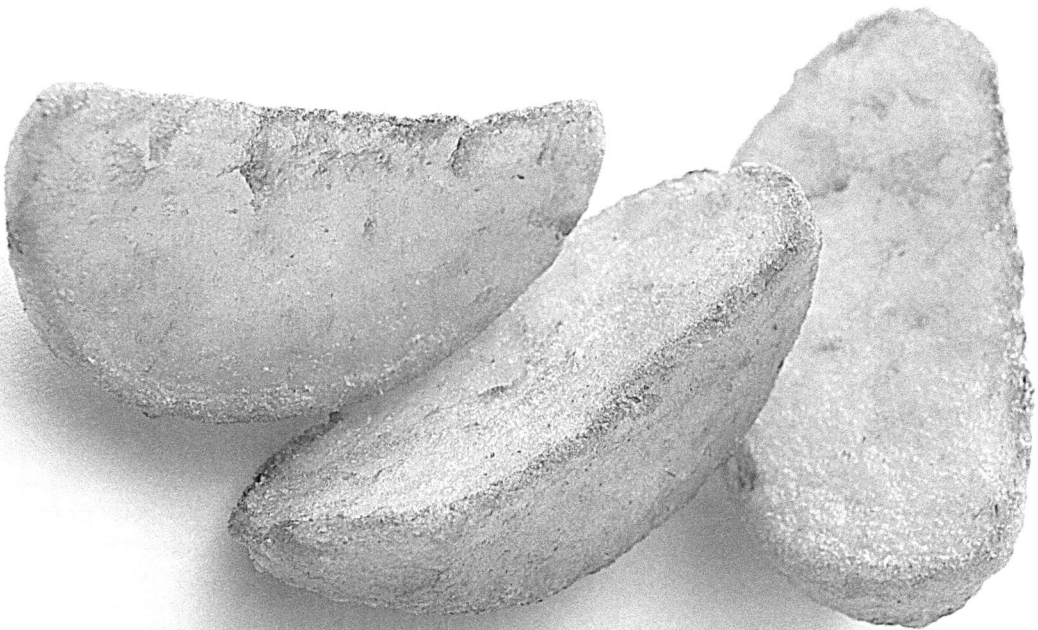

95

Fast food outlets use raw chips that are delivered cut and frozen – but before they are frozen the processing companies dunk the chips in either beef fat or palm oil so they won't stick together in the packet. So even before they reach the outlet, the chips already have a high content of saturated fat. Chips that are fried twice absorb almost twice as much fat as those fried once.

The frying oil can add insult to injury. Some outlets use solid 'blended edible vegetable oil' which proudly proclaims it has 'no cholesterol', but is silent about its likely content of nasty trans fat. In fact, no vegetable products contain cholesterol and it cannot be generated by frying. After years of lobbying, some of the major fast food outlets now use only frying fats with minimal trans fat. Ask if the outlet can assure you their frying fat has no trans fat. If not, shop elsewhere or make another choice.

The size of the serve is relevant. A medium serve of most fast food chips has about 21 g of fat and 1500 kJ. A similar serving of oven-fried chips (prepared at home) has about half as much fat. At least chips provide some dietary fibre.

FISH (AND CHIPS)

Fish is a healthy food, but when it is dipped into batter or crumbs and fried, the coating soaks up a lot of fat. Again, the frying fat is often solid frying oil, which can have a high content of trans fat, or one that contains either beef dripping or palm oil and thus will contribute saturated fat.

Most fish shops are happy to grill the fish, although 'grilling' usually means cooking the fish on a greased hot plate. The overall fat content is nonetheless low, and since the fish is more visible without its batter, most fish shops use a better quality fillet for grilling.

KEBABS

Shish kebabs are popular and potentially healthy with moderate quantities of meat (usually lamb or chicken) wrapped in a flatbread with tabbouli and hummus and felafel (chick pea patties) added. From a nutritional perspective, the major problem with most kebab wraps sold as fast food is their size. The average person really only needs half a serving. Some outlets will cut the kebab wrap in two, making this a reasonably healthy choice, although the salt content is usually high as salt is added to each of the ingredients. Tabbouli, hummus and felafel add a good content of dietary fibre and a range of vitamins and minerals.

PIES AND SAUSAGE ROLLS

According to Food Standards Australia New Zealand (FSANZ), the average Australian eats 12 meat pies a year and New Zealanders munch through 15 a year. Someone else eats mine – hopefully not babies or young children. FSANZ regards the meat pie as an 'iconic' food and has set a standard that they must contain at least 25 per cent meat. The meat can be beef, buffalo, camel, deer, goat, hare, lamb, mutton, pig, poultry or rabbit and can include any attached rind, fat, connective tissue, nerves, blood and blood vessels. If offal such as tongue, liver, spleen, kidney or tripe is added, it must be declared on the label along with the other ingredients. The rest of the pie is gravy, perhaps onion or occasionally some other vegetable, and its pastry crust. An average meat pie (175 g) has 2230 kJ, 35 g of fat (about half of it saturated or trans fat) and a high salt content. The meat contributes a small amount of iron and the pastry adds niacin (vitamin B3) and a small amount of dietary fibre. Depending on the pastry recipe, meat pies may also contain trans fat.

Sausage rolls are similarly high in kilojoules, fat and salt. New super-sized sausage rolls, reportedly developed for 'active men', are super high in kilojoules, fat, saturated fat and salt. An active man may need more kilojoules, but with 68 per cent of Australian men already carrying too much body fat, super-sized anything is inappropriate.

PIZZA

Like burgers, there is nothing nutritionally wrong with pizza. The Italian version, with bread dough topped with tomato, various vegetables drizzled with olive oil and a light hand with mozzarella, is delicious and healthy. Most fast food pizzas, however, feature fatty meats and lots of cheese and have few if any vegetables – but the main problem is the quantity consumed. As regulations come into play

97

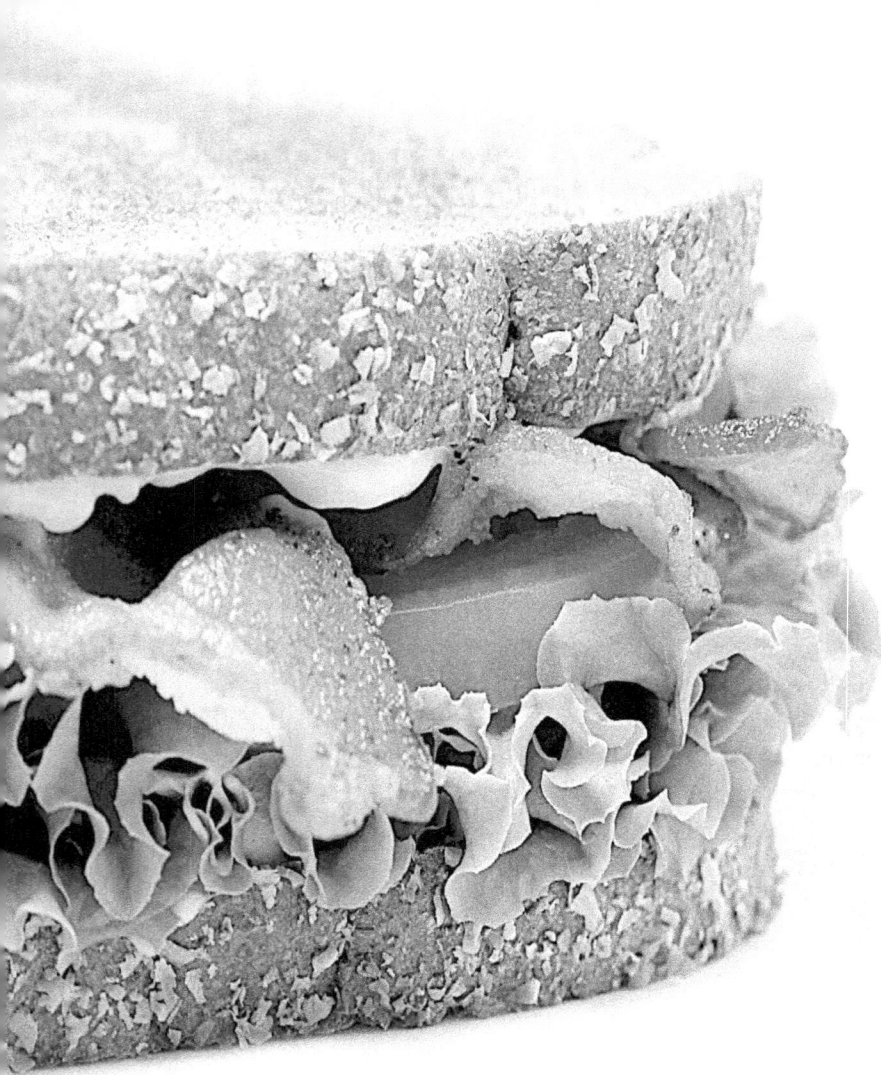

requiring kilojoule content to be prominently displayed, the values will probably be for a 'slice'. Many people eat six slices and wonder why their weight is increasing.

With pizza, go for quality products from independent restaurants, avoid processed meat toppings and check that the quantity of cheese is modest. And share!

SANDWICHES

Sandwiches made with baguettes, sliced bread, flat breads or rolls are a healthy choice. However, some fast food chains add lots of mayonnaise or sauces that contain fat and salt. Check the ingredients and the nutritional information usually available and choose items that include vegetables.

SUSHI

A healthy choice. Sushi and other Japanese 'finger foods' have become popular, especially with children. They are low in fat and many types containing nori (seaweed) are a good source of iodine, a mineral often lacking in the diet. The main problem is the high salt content of the soy sauce used for dipping. A quick dip will minimise the salt, and rice used for sushi is usually cooked without salt. Since sushi is eaten raw, clean premises for its preparation are important.

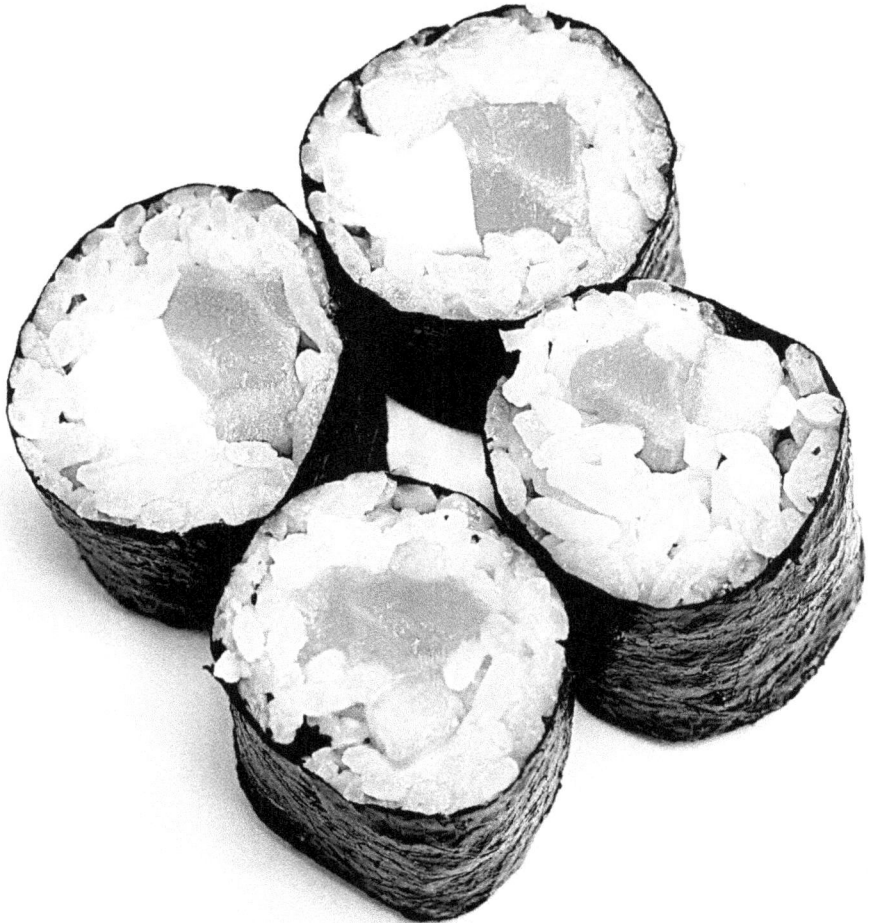

Fish
and other
seafoods
– catching the goodness

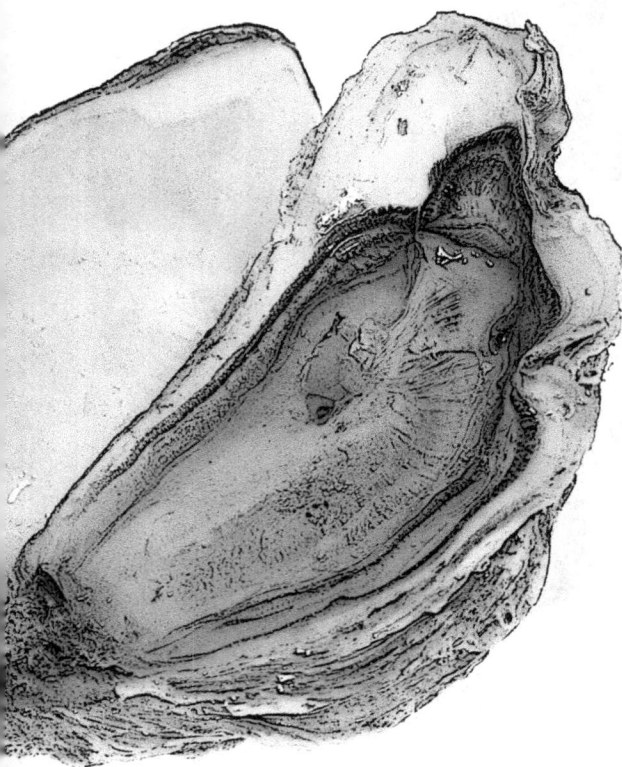

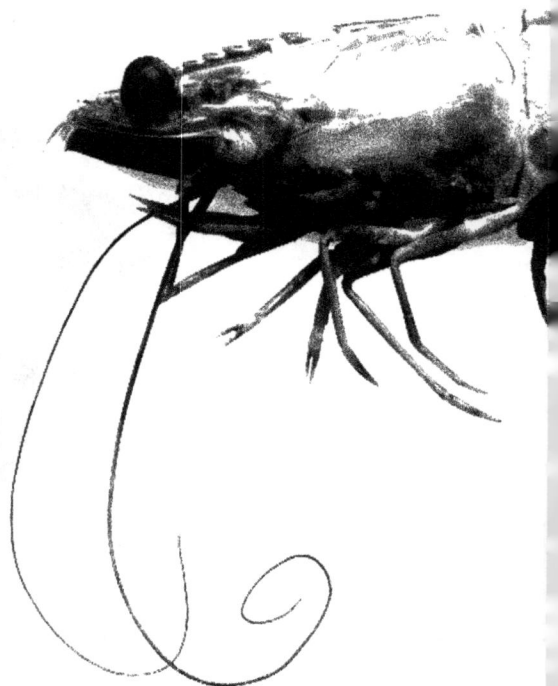

AUSTRALIAN FISH WERE ONCE damned by some authorities who thought that fish from warmer waters had less omega 3 fatty acids than those from cold waters. Studies of Inuit people in Greenland initially credited their lack of cardiovascular disease to a long-chain omega 3 fatty acid known as EPA (eicosapentaenoic acid), found in seal blubber, salmon, sardines and herrings. However, subsequent studies on the value of the fats in fish soon recognised the even greater value of another omega 3 fatty acid called DHA (docosahexaenoic acid). Analyses of Australian seafood (fish, crustaceans and molluscs) found they were an excellent source of DHA. (By convention, the omega 3 fatty acids are called omega 3s or omega 3 fats, but they are present, and active, in only milligram quantities, whereas the fats in most foods are measured in grams.) All Australian seafood, including shellfish, has enough omega 3s to be legally labelled as a 'good source' of these valuable fatty acids. The requirement for such a claim is that the food must have 60 mg of EPA + DHA. A food can have either 30 mg of EPA + DHA or 200 mg ALA (alpha linolenic acid) plus restricted levels of saturated and trans fatty acids and be labelled as a 'source'.

Where it all began

Professor Michael Crawford, of the Institute of Brain Chemistry and Nutrition at the University of North London, is one of the world's foremost authorities on omega 3 fatty acids. He believes that humans either had aquatic ancestors or developed their superior brain structure when they settled on estuaries and coastlines with ample access to rich sources of omega 3s from mussels, oysters, crabs and fish stranded in tidal pools, and that human brain capacity depended on pregnant women having ready access to foods rich in DHA. His theory gains strength from comparisons of the superb mental abilities and language skills of dolphins with the abilities of small-brained land-based animals such as the rhinoceros, elephant and hippopotamus. Unlike the dolphins with their omega 3-rich food sources, land animals usually have a diet low in omega 3s. Meat from grass-fed animals does contain small amounts of an omega 3 fatty acid called DPA (docosapentaenoic acid), which may have similar benefits to the omega 3s in seafood.

Why omega 3s are important

Before birth, omega 3s pass readily through the placenta to the foetus. After birth, babies get omega 3s from breast milk and they are incorporated into the retina and brain. Many studies show that babies who are breast-fed have higher IQ levels, even after correcting for factors such as differences in parents' socio-economic and educational status, the mother's health and behaviour before and during birth, and the infant's birth weight. Omega 3s also lead to sharper vision in the first few months of life, especially in pre-term infants.

Dozens of research studies support the value of omega 3s in reducing the risk of heart disease, type 2 diabetes and some types of cancer. Clinical trials have also shown a dramatic drop in second heart attacks in those who eat fish twice a week. Larger quantities do not seem to give greater benefits.

Current research is focusing on the benefits of DHA for the brain and its possible role in preventing dementia and treating depression. Mental health problems are rising, with predictions they will be one of the three major worldwide burdens of ill-heath by 2020. Many trials of omega 3s and depression are currently underway, but even before the results are in it would seem wise to recommend increases in consumption of foods rich in long-chain omega 3 fatty acids.

OMEGAS 3S AND BRAIN FUNCTION

Omega 3 fatty acids may have their greatest effects on brain function before birth and during infancy.

Early studies suggested that lower levels of the omega 3 fats EPA and DHA were associated with depression, mood swings and cognitive impairment in elderly people, but later, controlled studies using omega 3 supplements and a placebo have had mixed results. One study of young offenders at a maximum security institution reported that those given omega 3 supplements showed a 37 per cent reduction in violent offences during their time of incarceration. Other studies have reported less cognitive decline in elderly people given omega 3 supplements. For depression, the results are mixed, but any benefits appear to be related to EPA rather than DHA. Longer studies, including a 17-year follow-up in Australia and a large study of over 54000 women in the United

102

States, found that associations previously reported between omega 3s and depression did not hold up once other dietary and lifestyle factors were considered. Whether fish intake may be better than omega 3 supplements is not yet clear.

DIFFERENT KINDS OF OMEGA 3s

Foods such as linseeds (also called flaxseeds), canola, walnuts, oats and legumes, especially soy beans, contain an omega 3 fatty acid called alpha linolenic acid (ALA). Researchers are still unsure just how well ALA is converted to the longer chain omega 3s found ready-made in seafood. The brain's membranes use only DHA, so the body must convert ALA to this longer chain fatty acid. The process is obviously possible, since vegetarians have adequate quantities of DHA in the brain, but it may depend on avoiding large quantities of polyunsaturated vegetable oils since the fats in these oils compete for the same enzyme required to start converting ALA into DHA. For this reason, olive oil (which is low in polyunsaturated fat) is the preferred choice for vegetarians.

Other nutrients

As well as omega 3 fats, all types of seafood are an excellent source of protein and all are low in fats. Even 'fatty' fish have less total fat than lean meat. Like all animal foods, seafood contains ready-made cholesterol and prawns have higher levels than most other seafood. However, eating prawns is unlikely to raise blood cholesterol. High cholesterol levels occur when the body makes too much, which it does when the diet is high in saturated fat. Seafood (including prawns) has virtually no saturated fat.

Fish and seafood provide a rich load of other nutritional goodies, including iodine, zinc, iron and potassium, plus vitamins E, B2, B3, B6 (especially in crab, octopus and squid) and B12. Prawns, crab and oysters are also good sources of calcium. And if you happen to be marooned on a desert island with no fruit trees, octopus, squid and yabbies (freshwater crayfish) will supply more than enough vitamin C to protect you from scurvy. The nutritional virtues of seafood come with very few kilojoules. No one could ever grow fat on seafood unless it was always dipped in batter and fried. For zinc and iron, several types of shellfish easily outshine red meat, usually considered the richest source of these nutrients. Cockles, once sold to the poor of London along the wharves of the Thames, have 10 times as much iron as rump steak. Abalone also trumps steak by a factor of three, while mussels have four to five times as much iron as most cuts of red meat. Oysters score highly for iron, iodine, zinc and selenium.

Canned fish

Canned fish retain the nutrients of their fresh counterparts well. Fish canned in brine has higher levels of sodium from the added salt, while fish canned in oil has a higher kilojoule content. Whether fish is canned in water, brine or oil, some of the nutrients will escape into the liquid.

How much fish?

There is currently no recommended dietary intake for omega 3 fats, but dietary guidelines recommend one to two fish (or other seafood) meals a week. Unfortunately, humans have plundered fish stocks and polluted waters in many parts of the world, making this intake impossible for most people ever to achieve. Finding ways to preserve the marine food chain and developing sustainable methods of fish farming are vitally important. We can also expand the range of fish we use. Some species are discarded or used for cat food because they are not considered popular, sometimes because the fish is considered to be ugly! Some top chefs are trying to showcase the delicious dishes possible with less well-known fish species.

Climate change will have many effects on fishing, with some species threatened by changes in water temperature and currents, rising sea levels, increasing acidity of marine waters, increasing global temperature and changes in the amount and variability of rainfall. It is difficult

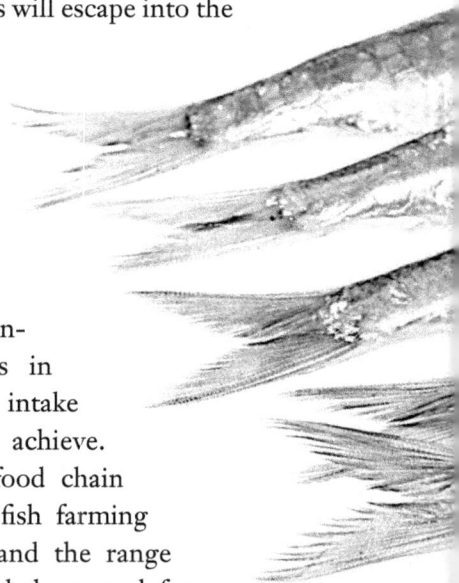

to give exact data on the species that are sustainable because the situation varies in different areas, and current management practices restrict the catch of some species in particular areas at particular times. Experts also fail to agree about which fish are vulnerable, although there is widespread agreement that shark, southern bluefin tuna and gemfish are currently overfished.

Aquaculture is increasing rapidly with ponds on land and in the ocean. Some farmed fish that are fed on fish meal pose problems for

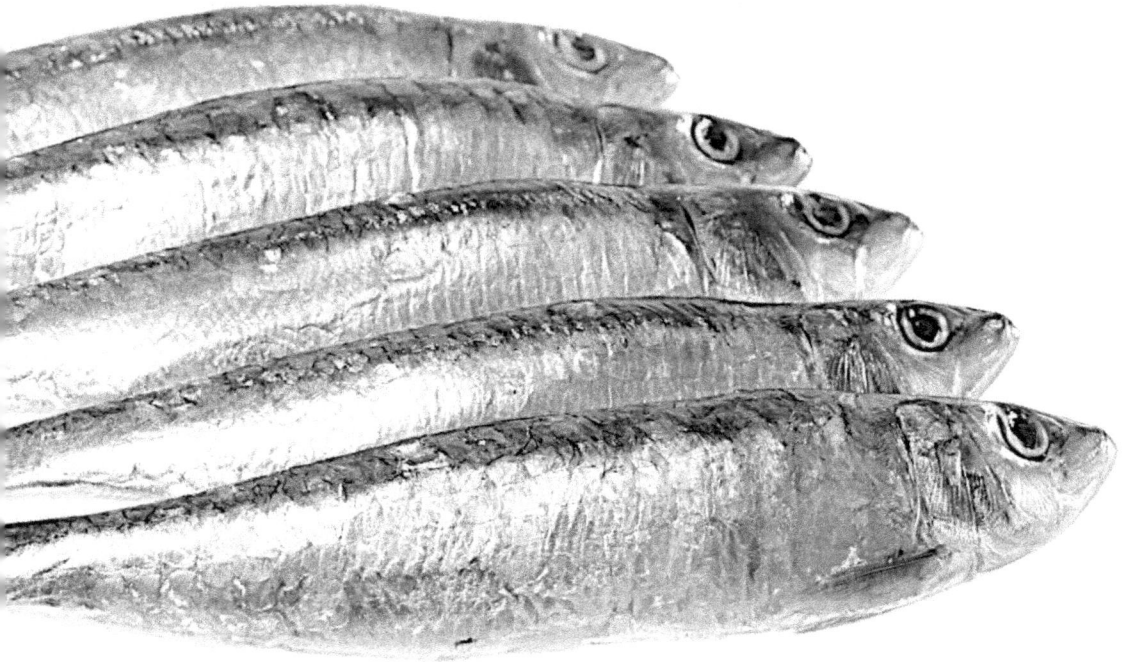

sustainability, but modern aquaculture is trying to avoid this with feed made up of waste from filleted fish, algae and land plants. Farming of oysters and prawns in Australia also takes pains to consider environmental factors. The Marine Stewardship Council certifies fisheries that conform to sustainability principles. Lists of sustainable fish are also available in a booklet or online from the Australian Marine Conservation Society <amcs.org.au>.

Would supplements be better?

Fish oil capsules make it possible to take in larger quantities of omega 3s, which can be useful in inflammatory conditions such as rheumatoid arthritis or for their drug-like effect in reducing blood fats called triglycerides.

Fish oil supplements can go 'off' easily. Always ensure they come from a reputable company with good laboratory and manufacturing facilities and ensure they are kept in a cool place. All omega 3 fats go rancid easily and rancid fats can cause disruption within the membranes that surround body cells. This is why fish doesn't keep well and canola oil and walnuts have a short shelf life. (Linseed oil goes rancid so rapidly that it's difficult to use it as a food, although its rapid oxidation makes it ideal to use on cricket bats and in paints.) In the case of not-so-fresh fish, your nose will alert you to rancidity, but rancidity may not be detectable when the fish oil is encased in a capsule. The dose of fish oil needed for a therapeutic effect also needs to be greater with capsules compared with eating fish. Researchers believe there may be other factors in fish that have a synergistic effect with their omega 3s.

Mercury fears

Fish and seafood absorb mercury, including mercury that occurs naturally in sea water and any arising from contamination. Fish from waters around Australia and New Zealand are not contaminated with mercury, but fish higher up the feeding chain will contain higher levels from natural sources. The quantities are not a problem for most people, but some restrictions are recommended for children under six and during pregnancy. These are:

- only 1 serve (150 g) a fortnight of swordfish, marlin or shark and no other fish that fortnight
- only 1 serve (150 g) a week of orange roughy (deep sea perch) or catfish and no other fish that week.

For all other fish and seafood, 2 to 3 serves a week are recommended.

Fruits
– how good are 'super fruits'?

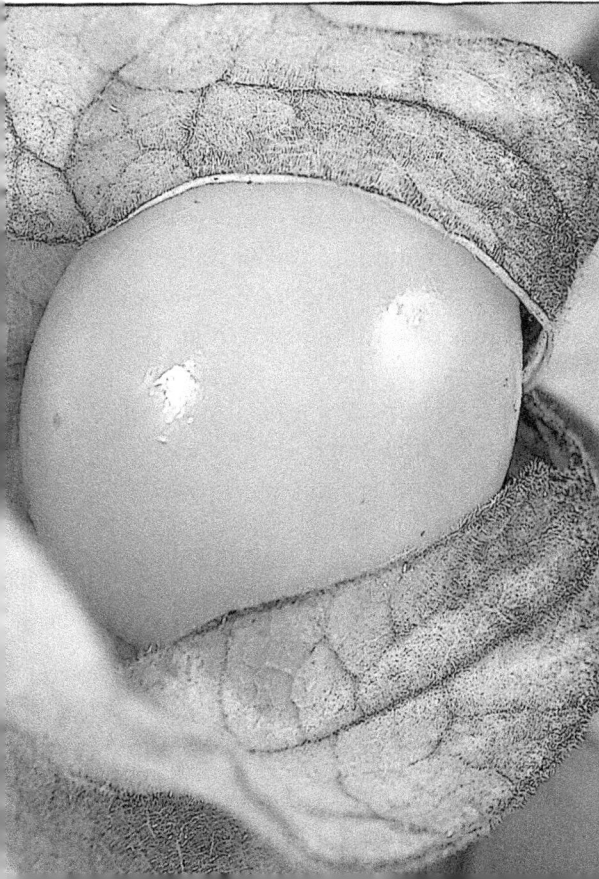

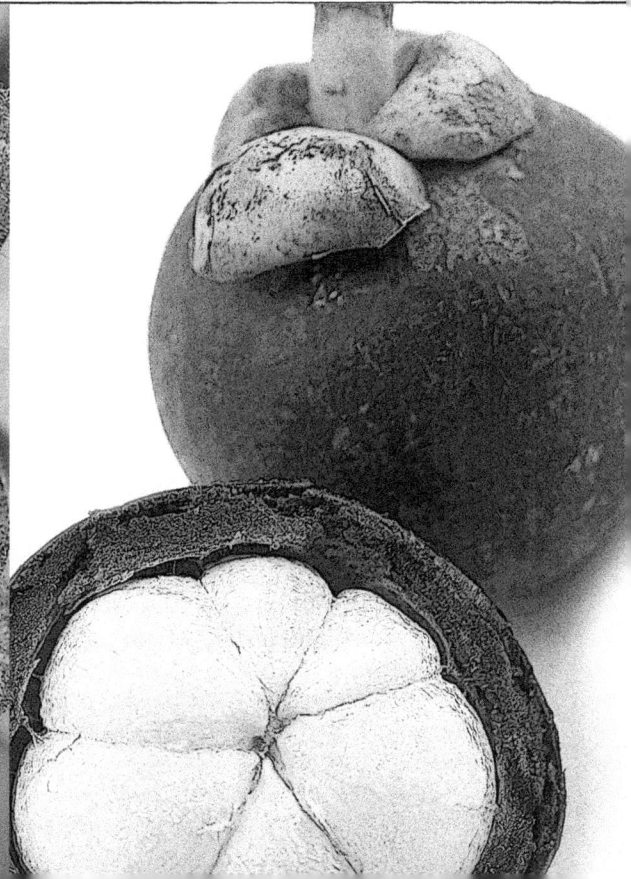

FRUITS ARE EXCELLENT FOODS, contributing vitamins, minerals and dietary fibre. Dietary guidelines recommend we have two servings of fruit a day because fruit helps reduce the risk of cardiovascular disease, diabetes and stroke. Those who eat fruit regularly are also less likely to be overweight, although this may not apply to those who regularly consume fruit juice.

Although fruit is so valuable, almost every week a magazine or newspaper features an article on the latest 'super fruit'. With no accepted definition for super foods, many suppliers make preposterous health claims, with some internet sites claiming their products will cure cancer, heart disease or other serious health problems. There are also claims that super fruits have anti-ageing benefits, referring to their use by some ancient culture, often in South America. Super foods are not always fruits, but fruits are favoured. Blueberries, cranberries and mangosteen share the limelight with more 'magic' goji berries (also known as wolfberries), noni fruit and açai and, quite recently, supplements containing African mango.

Blueberries

Like many purple and blue pigmented foods, blueberries are a source of polyphenols known as anthocyanins. The claim that blueberries have the highest level of these antioxidants has to compete against similar claims made for a range of other super fruits. In fact, fruits and vegetables contain over 400 anthocyanin compounds and different testing methods put different sources at or near the top. Disappointingly, research shows that those in berries are poorly available to the body, are extensively changed in the intestine and liver and are excreted in urine within 2–8 hours after consumption.

Blueberries are a delicious and nutritious fruit, a good source of vitamin C and dietary fibre, and notable for their content of an anthocyanin called cryptoxanthin. They are a worthwhile addition to the diet, but they don't really qualify as a super food.

Published studies include one observational study reporting fewer deaths from cardiovascular disease in women who ate blueberries and strawberries at least once a week, although another large study failed to confirm this. Various short-term studies giving extra berries, including blueberries, to small numbers of people, show some favourable effects on heart disease risk factors, but it is difficult to control for other factors or to separate the benefits from similar ones noted from an increased consumption of any fruit. The best advice is simply to enjoy them in season.

Cranberries

The bitterness of cranberries has curtailed their sales as a fresh berry and they are mostly sold in sugared and dried form, as a jelly or as juice. They do contribute vitamin C and dietary fibre, but their bitterness means they are usually consumed dried and sweetened or in juices. Some studies have found that a compound in cranberry juice can help reduce the incidence of urinary tract infections. The most recent well-controlled trial among women with urinary tract infections concluded that after six months, those consuming 250 mL of cranberry juice twice a day had no decrease in incidence of a second infection compared with those drinking a placebo juice. Earlier positive trials suffered from large dropout rates due mainly to a dislike of the taste of the juice, and no results were found in men of comparable age to the women in these studies, in children or in elderly men and women. More studies may clear up the confusion, but cranberries are best classified as fruits – not super fruits.

Incaberries

Sometimes 'super' status comes with a new name, possibly to emphasise some exotic ancestry. This has occurred with *Phyalis peruviana* (commonly known as Cape gooseberries or golden berries), now being marketed as dried 'incaberries', complete with claims of being gluten free (of course they are, because gluten occurs only in wheat, rye, triticale and barley!) and having super high antioxidant levels. Cape gooseberries hail from South America and were planted by early settlers in South Africa and Australia. They now grow wild in many parts of both countries.

A member of the nightshade family, incaberries are related to tomatoes, eggplant and potatoes and are a good source of vitamin C (when fresh, but some is lost when they are dried), beta carotene and dietary fibre. They also contain some iron. Claims that they contain vitamin

109

B12 and thus 'support cellular metabolism' are false since this vitamin is found only in animal foods. Grubs in the berries, perhaps?

Mangosteen

Sometimes available in fruit shops in Australia, the mangosteen is a delicious-tasting fruit from South-East Asia that also grows well in tropical parts of Australia. Claims about super fruit status refer not to the sweet white fleshy segments but to the thick rind (or pericarp) that covers the fruit. The pericarp is a source of xanthones, which enthusiasts claim to be 'the most powerful antioxidants found in nature'. (Another range of naturally occurring xanthones has previously been used as insecticides.)

Mangosteen fruit is supposed to protect against breast cancer, liver cancer and leukaemia, as well as having anti-inflammatory and anti-histamine properties. The xanthones from the rind are supposed to have beneficial effects for heart disease and high blood pressure, to prevent clots and relax blood vessels. Enthusiasts also claim that mangosteen protects against various bacterial and viral infections, strengthens the immune system and helps wounds heal.

Published studies mostly involve laboratory tests of extracts of mangosteen rind with researchers identifying the active compounds within the rind. One small study gave an extract containing mangosteen, aloe vera, green tea and multivitamins to human volunteers and reported some bioavailability of two B complex vitamins and a mild and transitory antioxidant effect, possibly from a substance in the mangosteen. Other studies have used concentrated xanthone extracts and reported they may kill particular cells. This is not surprising considering their past use in insecticides, but it's a far cry from making health claims for mangosteen – incidentally, the flesh doesn't contain the xanthones found in the rind. At this stage, the magic is missing.

Goji berries

These bright red-orange berries, native to many parts of China and the Himalayan region, were first marketed on the internet, often as a juice. The dried berries are now available in supermarkets and are moving from the health food aisle into some mueslis and confectionery bars.

110

A long string of unverifiable claims is made for goji berries. They are claimed to lower blood pressure, prevent cancer, maintain healthy cholesterol levels, help with weight loss, balance blood sugar and manage diabetes, relieve headaches and symptoms of menopause, assist vision and banish a chronic dry cough. If you have no obvious health problems, you may be more interested in their supposed ability to improve energy, memory and fertility, strengthen the legs and stimulate the release of human growth hormone so you'll look and feel younger. Many of these claims appear with glowing testimonials from supposedly satisfied users. One site has several doctors attesting to the berries' powers for themselves and their patients, with claims they have cured problems ranging from reflux and restless legs to cancer.

When searching for published medical evidence, you find nothing under 'goji', but there are some studies listed under the alternative names *Lycium barbarum* and English wolfberry. None match the extravagant claims listed above. One study of 50 Chinese people (one of the authors was a seller of a goji juice product) claimed that those in the study taking goji juice produced higher levels of the body's normal antioxidant compounds.

Like many fruits and vegetables, these berries are a source of zeaxanthin, one of the two carotenoids which have been associated with reducing the risk of age-related macular degeneration. A small German study with 12 participants reported that the zeaxanthin in wolfberries is absorbed into the bloodstream, so there is at least a possibility of some benefit for the eyes, although proof of absorption is not quite the same as a clinical effect. Zeaxanthin is found in greatest abundance in kale, spinach, rocket and dark green Asian vegetables and is also present in broccoli, sweet corn, persimmons, oranges and mandarins.

Claims that goji berries have 500 times as much vitamin C as oranges, more amino acids than bee pollen, and provide a wide range of vitamins and minerals, are preached to potential buyers as though they were gospel. No published analysis supports the claims. There is also no evidence the berries assist weight loss.

In Chinese medicine, the bark of the *Lycium barbarum* shrub is reputed to have benefits in reducing blood pressure, although no controlled studies appear to have examined this. Future studies may find

111

some clinical value for goji/wolfberries, but until such studies are published in reputable journals, it may be more important to note that the berries can cause adverse reactions in those taking the blood-thinning medication warfarin.

Noni fruit

Also called Indian mulberry or cheese fruit, the noni (*Morinda citrifolia*) grows in some Pacific Island countries and parts of Asia. Noni juice is sold mostly through multi-level marketing schemes. Some sellers achieved public prominence a few years ago when the Australian Competition and Consumer Commission issued prosecutions for claims that their juice products could cure diabetes and cancer. Since then, internet claims have been somewhat more subdued, alleging only that the product supports the immune system to strengthen the body's natural ability to fight disease and infection, assists digestion to improve absorption of nutrients at the cellular level, increases mental clarity and attention span, supports the heart and joints, or provides for greater recovery from sports exertion. Noni products are also said to bring shine to the hair and a glow to the skin.

Among the published material on noni fruit, one study found no fertility problems in mice given noni juice. Several others list authors with obvious conflicts of interest, although that criticism can be levelled at many scientific papers. It is unacceptable, however, for a scientific paper to note (in passing) that the fruit 'has been reported to have a broad range of health benefits for cancer, infection, arthritis, diabetes,

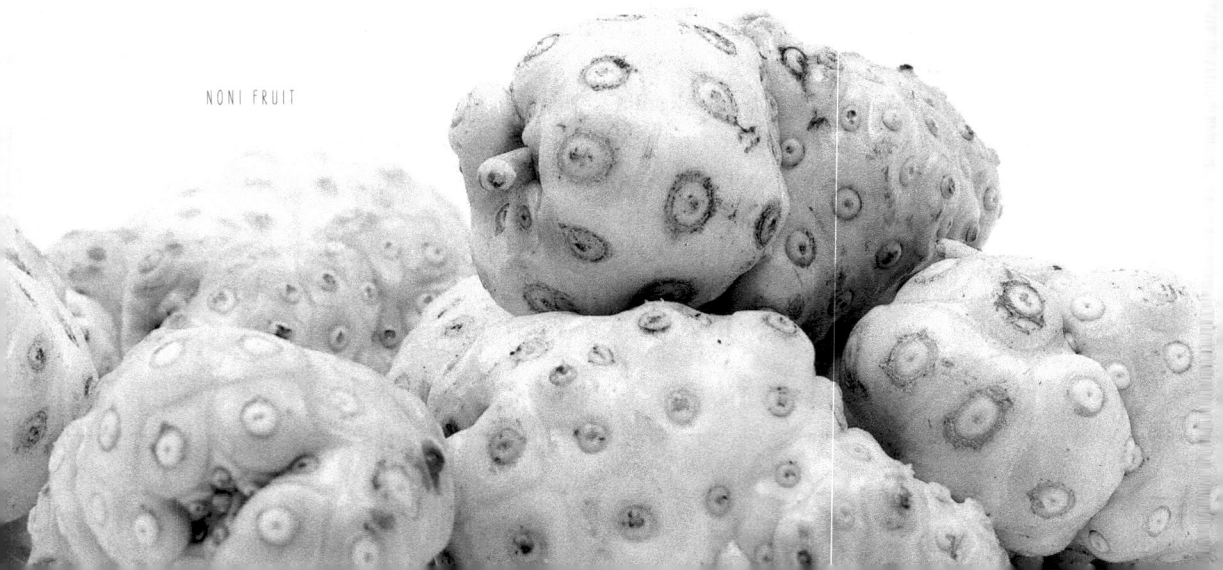

NONI FRUIT

asthma, high blood pressure and pain' without providing accompanying references. It is also unacceptable to extrapolate from such studies to suggest that noni juice might improve fecundity and foetal health and to dismiss contrary reports on the basis that the purity of some noni juice is not 'authenticated'.

Noni has a long history of use in traditional medicine. The leaves and roots appear to contain some pharmacologically active compounds. One laboratory study from China has shown that compounds extracted from the roots may have some activity against cancer cells. A Japanese study reports that a compound isolated and extracted from noni root may exert anti-inflammatory effects in mice. A compound extracted from dried noni fruit is also reported to reduce reflux-induced oesophagitis in rats while juice fermented for up to 10 weeks is reported to have some (small) beneficial effects in diabetic rats. Compounds that have been identified in noni juice include saponins, triterpenes, steroids, flavonoids and cardiac glycosides, and various companies are trying to isolate sufficient quantities of some of these for use in pharmaceutical preparations. Extracting and purifying compounds from plants is a basic part of pharmacology, but it is not valid to extrapolate from that to assume equally potent effects from consuming the leaves, roots, flowers or fruit of a plant. Many compounds that exhibit potent biological activity are present in their plants of origin at very low levels of concentration.

Independent (that is, those not funded by sellers of noni juice) human studies of noni juice are rare. One from Thailand claims that an extract of dried noni fruit (at high dose) can help prevent nausea and vomiting after surgery. There have, however, been several reports of severe liver damage after taking large quantities of noni juice.

Noni juice is expensive (about \$35–\$50 a litre), although usually cheaper than goji juice (up to \$70 a litre). But then goji juice claims to have four times the 'life force' of noni juice! As most people rate the taste of noni as unpleasant, potential customers should check what they are paying for. Many products are extensively diluted with a more pleasant tasting (and much cheaper) product such as apple or grape juice. To avoid the taste problem, one company now puts noni juice into capsules, and also sells it dried and powdered, combined with inulin, Siberian ginseng, soy lecithin, pumpkin seed, spinach, calcium, green tea extract, cinnamon, globe artichoke, cranberry, rose-hips, flaxseed, liquorice root, milk thistle, potassium, bilberry and ginger, in a soy powder base. Another sells a special noni formula for horses.

Until the benefits are proven in human studies, the anecdotal reports of cures and testimonials from untraceable 'satisfied users' or members of marketing schemes offering to make you a millionaire are not proof the products are effective. At least their high price makes it unlikely that the juice products will be consumed in excess.

Açai fruit

This dark purple fruit that looks like a very small grape with a large seed comes from a tall slender palm (*Euterpe oleracea*) that grows in swamps and floodplains in Central and South America. Contrary to claims made by those selling the berries, the palm is common and widely distributed, since birds and rodents alike appreciate its prolific crop of berries. In Brazil, the juice is squeezed from the açai berries

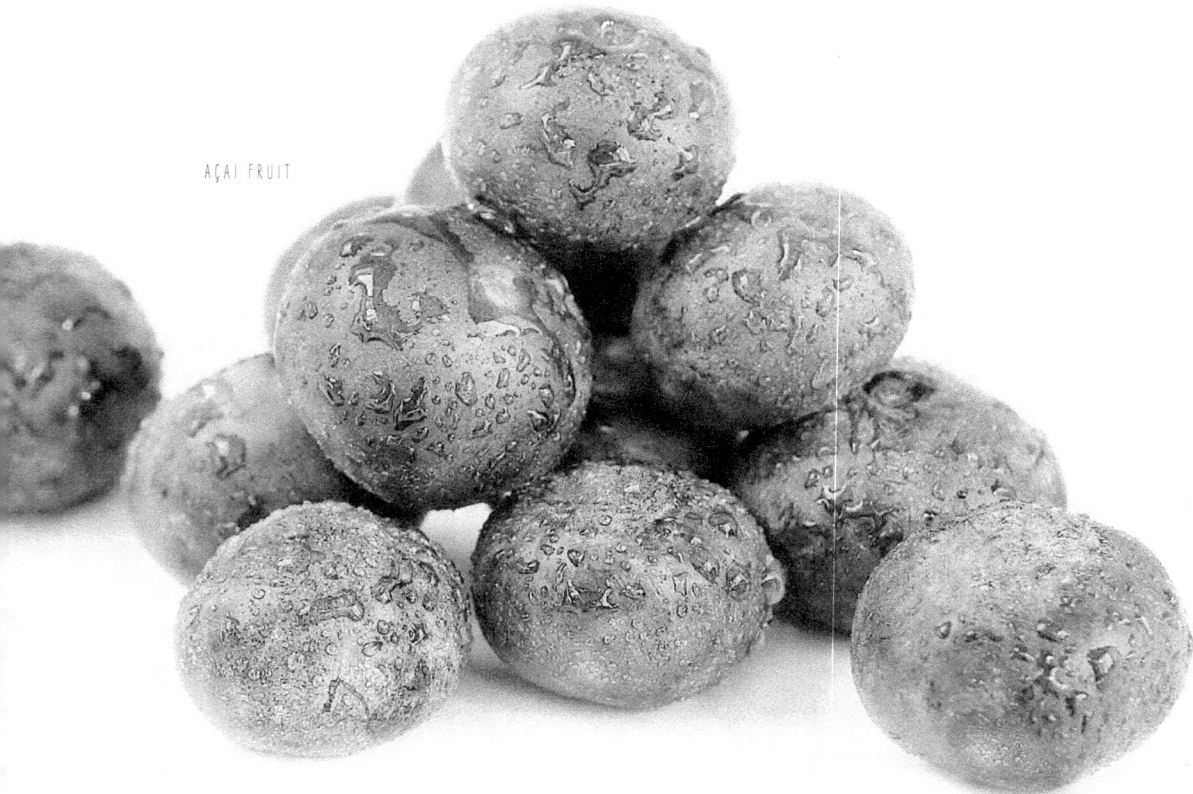

AÇAI FRUIT

after soaking and, unlike the juices of some other super fruits, is considered delicious. The juice may be mixed with extra sugar and sometimes with tapioca flour to make a refreshing drink, and the pulp may be mixed with sugar or honey and tapioca or other grains. In Australia, açai is mostly sold as a juice or a supplement of freeze-dried powder by multi-level marketers who describe it as 'a gift of the gods'.

In the quantities likely to be consumed, the nutrient content is unremarkable and not dissimilar to other fruits. Claims of a very high content of dietary fibre and protein mistakenly use the values from an analysis of freeze-dried açai powder and assume it also applies to the berries.

Açai berries do contain beta sitosterol, a compound that has the potential to reduce the absorption of cholesterol. One study found that dried açai pulp reduced 'bad' LDL cholesterol in rats fed a diet designed to increase their blood cholesterol levels.

The berries also contain a range of polyphenols (see Antioxidants, page 34) including anthocyanins (which produce much of the pigmented colouring) and a range of phenolics. These compounds have potential antioxidant action, but some studies show poor absorption and degradation with storage or heat. Again, the actual content is probably unremarkable. Levels of most of the polyphenols are lower in freeze-dried açai powders and claims that açai has the highest antioxidant level of any food don't fit with published research.

Internet sellers of açai products allege their products promote better sleeping patterns, mental clarity, are good for glaucoma and macular degeneration, reduce signs of ageing (including loss of neurological function) and help with weight loss. None of these claims is proven. A small pilot study in which 10 overweight people were given 100 g of açai pulp twice a day for 30 days found no drop in weight or blood pressure and although the researchers claimed some fall in blood glucose and cholesterol levels, the values were so varied that no conclusion was possible. In prosecuting some companies selling açai products for internet scams, the US Federal Trade Commission notes that companies have no proof for weight loss. Don't be tempted to give credit card details to a company offering free samples of açai for just a small shipping fee. It's a case of buyer beware! There is no magic here.

Grains
– go for the goodness of the whole

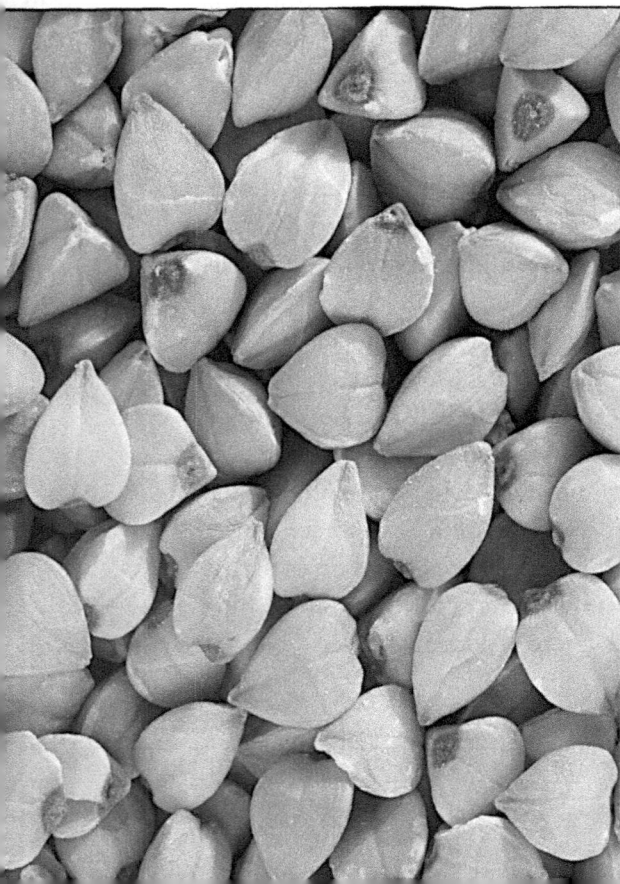

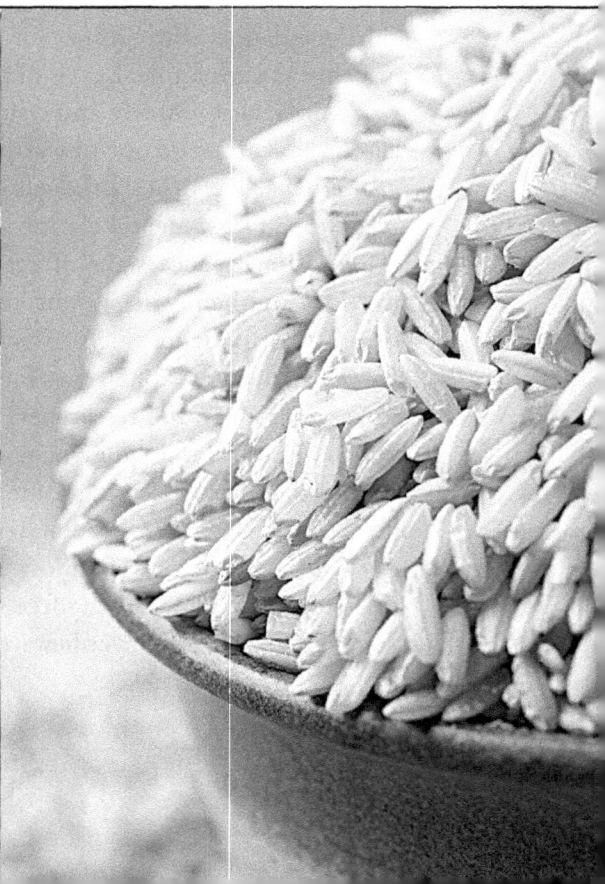

IT'S HARD TO THINK OF FOODS that have been more important to human history and health than grains. New techniques that allow archeo-botanists to measure minute changes in pollens and ancient cereal grains have established that our ancestors used cereal grains well before farming began and much earlier than has been previously assumed. The inhabitants of Ohallo II (in areas now included in Israel) made the seeds of wild grasses a major part of their diet at least 19 000 years ago. Archeological evidence now shows that our ancestors congregated where grasses grew and gradually moved to cultivating them as a reliable source of food, thousands of years before they began to farm animals. It is fair to say that cultivation of grains led to a transition for humans from a nomadic way of life to the development of settlements, towns and cities.

All grains are nutritionally valuable, especially as they can be stored for long periods without losing their nutrients. While we usually think of grains as a source of starchy carbohydrate, they also provide protein, dietary fibre, and many minerals and vitamins. Grains provide about 27 per cent of the average Australian adult's protein intake, much higher than the contribution from dairy products.

Whole grains have many health benefits, reducing the risk of cardio-vascular disease and some cancers. They are also filling and thus valuable for people needing to lose weight. Definitions vary, but generally the term 'whole grain' means that the bran, germ and endosperm are present in the proportions of the original grain.

Whole grains contain compounds called phytates which can bind minerals such as calcium and iron, making them less available to the body. The phytates bind only some of the minerals present in the grain and have no effect on those from other foods that may be eaten at the same meal. Yeast added to bread dough, and the action of wild yeasts in sourdough breads, causes the phytates to release their hold on minerals. In practice, the binding effect of phytates in whole grains is only a problem in places where diets are marginal and unleavened bread is the norm.

When grains are refined, the bran and germ are removed, leaving the endosperm. As the germ and bran contain much of the dietary fibre, vitamins and minerals, from a nutritional perspective refined grains are inferior products. Since fibre delays the time taken for foods to be digested, refined grains are digested much more rapidly. For those with diabetes,

117

the higher glycaemic index (GI) of refined grains means a more rapid influx of glucose into the bloodstream. Wholemeal bread made from a recombination of white flour, wheatgerm and bran also has a higher GI than bread made from ground whole grains of wheat.

Which grains?

The most commonly consumed grains in Australia are wheat and rice, but some of the other grains that are also available have much to offer.

AMARANTH

Different types of amaranth find use either as a vegetable or a grain. Although now hailed as an exotic new product, the Aztecs cultivated and enjoyed it for thousands of years, making full use of the fact that it grows in quite poor soils. Nutritionally, amaranth grain comes close to the top of the class with a high content of protein, iron and zinc, as well as providing calcium and dietary fibre. It has no gluten and can be used as a breakfast cereal or as a nutritious substitute for rice.

BARLEY

Originally grown in northern Africa and South-East Asia, from about 3500 to 2300 BC, barley was used as one of the basic units of the ancient Sumerian measuring system. Length, volume and mass were measured from a gur, a theoretical standard cube that could be filled with barley, wheat, water or oil. Barley is a tough grain and can withstand dryness, frost and poor soils. It is still eaten in many Middle Eastern countries, usually ground into a flour to make flatbreads. Tibetan Buddhist monks carry a bag of barley flour to mix with yak's milk and cook into a porridge called tsampa. If cooking facilities are not available, small balls of the dough are eaten raw.

Barley is 'pearled' by removing its outer brown layers. This removes some of its fibre and nutrients, but it remains nutritious, with higher levels of most nutrients than rice. It cooks slowly but is a useful addition to soups or casseroles. Barley water is a traditional remedy for kidney problems but modern research shows that the soluble fibres called beta glucans in barley and barley water are more likely to be beneficial for bowel health. Barley contains gluten, although less than wheat, and this

118

means that barley breads tend to be heavy. The carbohydrates in barley are digested slowly, giving it a low GI value. Lemon barley water is an old-fashioned drink that is used as a tonic in folk medicine.

BUCKWHEAT

Although it is the fruit of a herbaceous plant rather than a true cereal, buckwheat is usually classified with cereals on the basis of its starchy carbohydrates. Originating in Asia and used in China for making bread, in European countries it is steamed or made into a porridge. It contains no gluten and is used in mixed flours to make gluten-free pasta, bread, and pancakes commonly known as blini.

BULGUR

Made from ground, cooked dried wheat and popular in Eastern Europe and the Middle East, bulgur is familiar to most people as the grain in tabbouli. It is quick to prepare: pour boiling water over the grain (two cups of water to one cup of bulgur), cover tightly and leave to stand for about 10 minutes, when the water will be absorbed. Either eat it hot in place of rice, or for tabbouli cool and mix with lots of chopped parsley, diced cucumber and tomato and some lemon juice and extra virgin olive oil. Bulgur is a good source of iron, protein, dietary fibre and vitamins of the B group and vitamin E.

CORN

Native to Mexico, corn has been the staple food for the Indians of South and Central America for thousands of years. Different varieties of corn are now grown for human and animal food and it is used as a vegetable and a grain. Ground corn is an ingredient in some breads and pastas (including gluten-free varieties) in Australia and polenta has become popular, made from either white or yellow corn. Many more uses are made of corn in the United States, where it is fed to chickens (making their flesh yellow), used for corn syrup, corn oil and as a base material in making bourbon whisky.

Some varieties of corn are excellent for popping. Corn has both protein and starch when heated, the small amount of moisture present causes the starch to gelatinise. As the temperature inside the grain increases, the water expands and exerts pressure on the protein so that the kernel bursts open, allowing the centre portion (the endosperm) to expand. At the same time, the gelatinised starch dries, leaving a crisp popped kernel of corn. When popped in a large saucepan using a small amount of oil, or made with a hot-air popper, popcorn has a low level of fat and is a good source of dietary fibre. Commercially popped corn usually has a high level of fat plus the disadvantage of added salt.

Sweet corn is a variety of corn with a higher content of natural sugars. It is picked when the kernels are at their soft, immature stage and is usually included as a vegetable rather than a grain. High in dietary fibre and slowly-digested carbohydrate, sweet corn is also a source of iron, folate and vitamin E. Canned corn retains its nutrients and is available without added salt.

COUSCOUS

Generally made from semolina, the central part of the wheat grain, couscous can also be made from millet. Popular in North African countries, mainly as an accompaniment to dishes featuring chick peas, vegetables and spices, couscous is also used as a dessert, often mixed with honey or sugar, cinnamon and pomegranate juice. It is now common in Australia and many European countries. As well as its carbohydrate, it provides dietary fibre, some iron and niacin (vitamin B3).

MILLET

This hardy grain is a popular seed for birds, but was once the main cereal in Europe, parts of Africa and Asia, and is still widely used in India, Ethiopia, Russia and Egypt. Before rice took over, millet was also a staple grain in China and remains popular in northern China. Because it has no gluten, millet does not produce good bread, but it can be used in flatbreads and is the major ingredient in injera, the national bread of Ethiopia. It can also be used in stews and soups, or mixed with various legumes. It is a good source of dietary fibre, vitamins of the B group and some minerals.

OATS

Much of the research extolling the nutritional virtues of whole grains in reducing the risk of cardiovascular disease and some cancers refers to oats. Native to Central Europe, but later a staple in Scotland, Ireland and

120

the north of England, oats have traditionally been eaten as a porridge or added to bread and biscuits. They also form the basis of muesli, a highly nutritious mixture of oats, nuts, seeds and dried fruit. As consumption of oats has declined in Scotland, so has the health of the population.

Oats are a valuable source of soluble fibres called beta glucans, and their protein content is almost as high as that of eggs. Although oats contain more fat than most grains, it is unsaturated fat and a good source of essential fatty acids. They also provide iron, zinc, potassium and other minerals (including manganese), vitamin E and several of the B complex vitamins. Oats do not contain gluten, but some people with coeliac disease also have an adverse reaction to the protein in oats. Oats which are grown or processed near wheat may become contaminated with wheat grains.

Rolled oats are made by flattening the oat. Quick-cooking oats are made by cutting the oats into finer flakes; there is no loss of nutritional value, but a slightly higher GI value results because they can be digested a little faster. More expensive brands of oats ensure that no bits of husk remain, but have no other advantages. Oat bran is finely milled and may not retain the endosperm, thus reducing its content of vitamin E and soluble fibre.

A typical bowl of oat porridge has no more kilojoules than a bowl of a light, puffed or popped breakfast cereal. Cooking oats in a bowl in the microwave eliminates the need to wash a saucepan. Oats can also be eaten raw.

QUINOA

Originally grown in the Andes, quinoa was the staple food of the Incas. It is now grown in Australia. The most nutritious of all grains, quinoa has a high content of protein and dietary fibre, as much iron as meat, and scores well for zinc, magnesium, potassium and vitamins B1, B2, B3, B6, folate and vitamin E. It can be cooked like rice and used in similar ways. It is also popular with fruit as a breakfast porridge. Quinoa has no gluten and is a top choice for those with coeliac disease.

RICE

Although rice has been a staple in China and many Asian countries for at least 5000 years, scholars now believe this grain originated in India. Rice

121

is usually grown in paddies which are flooded with water until the grain is ready to ripen. The paddies are then drained and the rice is picked and harvested by machines. Small fish are often raised in rice paddies in Asia and later dried and powdered for use in sauces that are a major source of calcium.

Brown rice is the most nutritious form of rice. White rice has had the bran removed by abrasive milling and this also removes some of the dietary fibre, minerals and vitamins. Parboiled rice is partially cooked with its bran layer and some of the nutrients pass into the grain. The bran is removed after the rice is dried. Wild rice is not really a rice, but a tall aquatic grass which grows in China, Japan and the Great Lakes region of North America. It is difficult to cultivate, is more expensive than rice and has a nutty flavour.

If rice contains broken grains, some starch leaks and makes the rice gluggy when it is cooked. Sticky or glutinous rice is available in purple-black or white varieties and is popular in some parts of Asia for sweets. Basmati rice was originally grown in the foothills of the Himalayas and has a slightly aromatic flavour. Arborio and carnaroli rice absorb much more water without going soggy and are used for risotto. Doongara rice was developed in Australia and is digested more slowly, giving it a lower glycaemic index. This can be useful for those with diabetes.

Claims that rice is fattening do not fit with the fact that when rice dominates the diet in Asian countries, obesity is rare. As Asian populations adopt a western-style diet with less rice and more fat, sugar and animal products, obesity and type 2 diabetes increases.

When rice is cooked by the absorption method (two cups of water for each cup of rice), some of the starch escapes digestion in the small intestine and passes to the bowel, where it is broken down by bacteria in a similar way to dietary fibre. This may help explain the low incidence of bowel cancer in most Asian populations, even though the fibre content of their diet is low.

RYE

Rye is mostly used in breads, either with wheat in light rye loaves or on its own in the dark and heavy rye breads popular in Germany, Scandinavia and many Eastern European countries. Rye flour contains gluten and cannot be used by those with coeliac disease. Wholegrain rye is an excellent source of dietary fibre as well supplying protein, iron and smaller quantities of other minerals and vitamins.

SORGHUM

The staple grain of Africa and parts of Asia, sorghum is also called kaffir corn, Guinea corn or African corn. Young sorghum plants contain a high level of prussic acid that is poisonous to cattle (and humans). As the plant matures and is cut and dried, the prussic acid content is dissipated and the plant can be used for cattle feed. For human consumption, sorghum is usually ground into a flour that can be used in gluten-free products. It is high in protein, iron, niacin (vitamin B3) and dietary fibre.

SPELT

An old variety of wheat, grown in Europe at least 9000 years ago, spelt is now being grown in Australia. Its increasing popularity is partly because it requires less fertiliser and pesticide than other forms of wheat, making it potentially 'greener'. Contrary to popular belief, spelt contains gluten and is not suitable for people with coeliac disease.

TRITICALE

This grain was developed in the 1960s as a hybrid of rye and wheat, designed to grow in similar conditions to rye, but to contain more gluten to improve the quality of bread. Triticale is not suitable for gluten-free diets, but provides protein, iron, potassium and vitamins of the B complex.

WHEAT

Wheat was first cultivated in western parts of Asia, and has been milled since at least 4000 BC. The Egyptians used stone grinding wheels to crack the grains and mixed the resulting meal with water to make flat cakes, baked on hot stones. Wheat is now grown in many parts of the world and is ideal for bread because its high content of gluten provides structure to the loaf. Hard wheats used for bread and pasta have the highest content of protein and gluten, soft wheats used for cakes and biscuits the lowest.

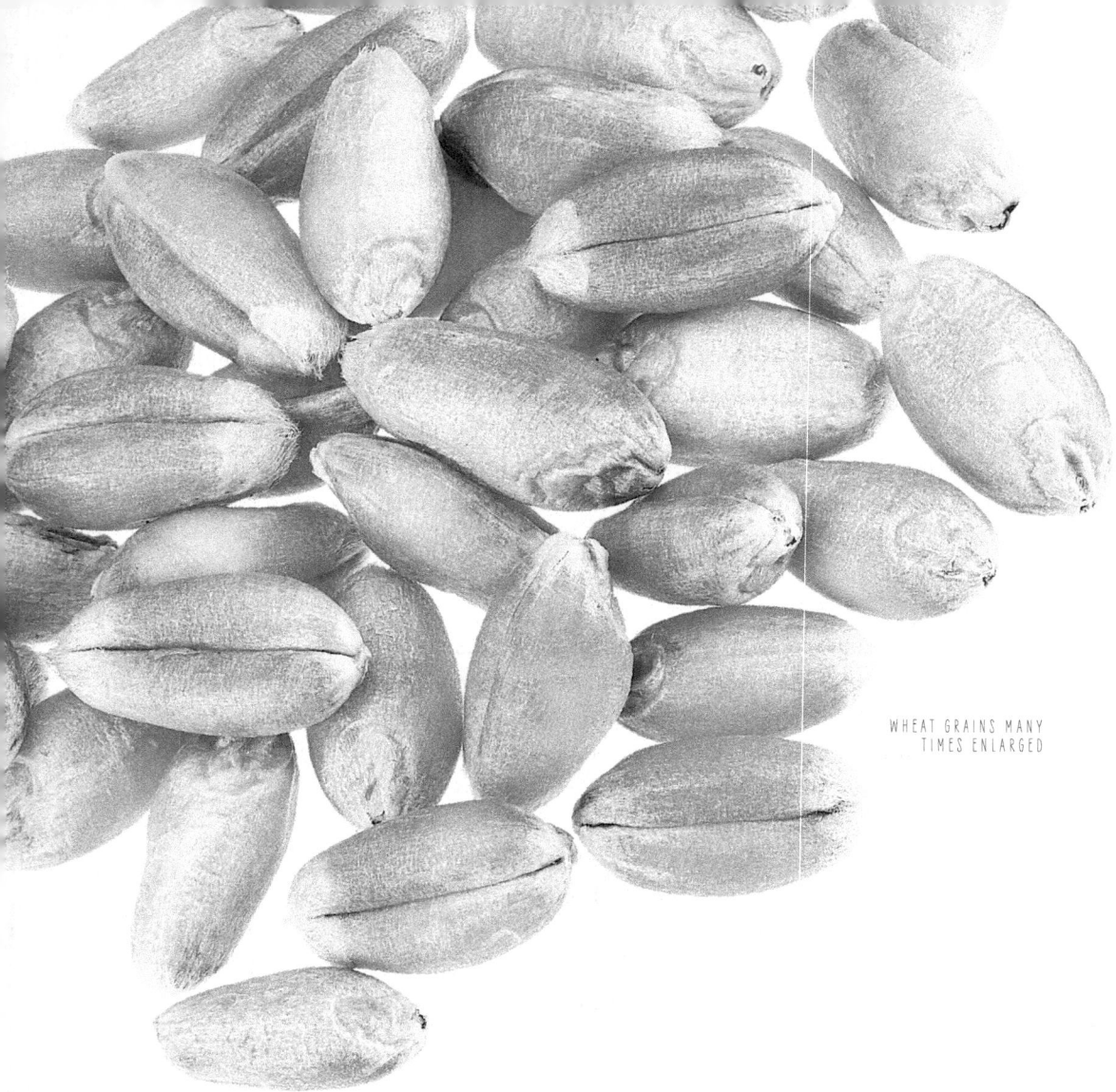

Wheat is mainly sold as wholemeal or white flour. Wholemeal flour is a source of protein, vitamins of the B group, vitamin E, protein, dietary fibre and a range of minerals. White flour has lower levels of nutrients, but bread-making flour in Australian is fortified with thiamin (vitamin B1) and folic acid (another vitamin of the B complex). White flour is no longer bleached.

Wheat is also used to make pasta, breakfast cereals and a range of baked goods whose nutritional value depends on what else is added.

124

Meat
– when less is more

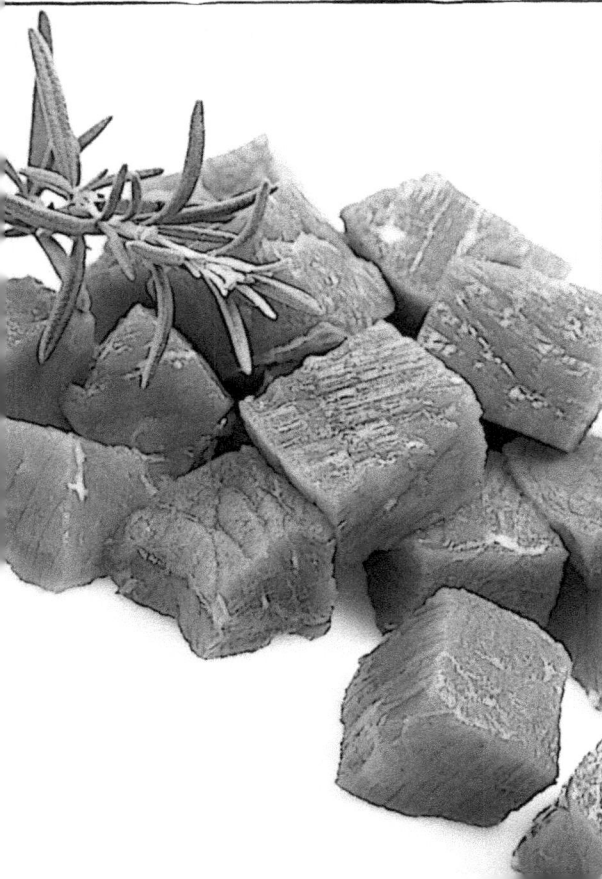

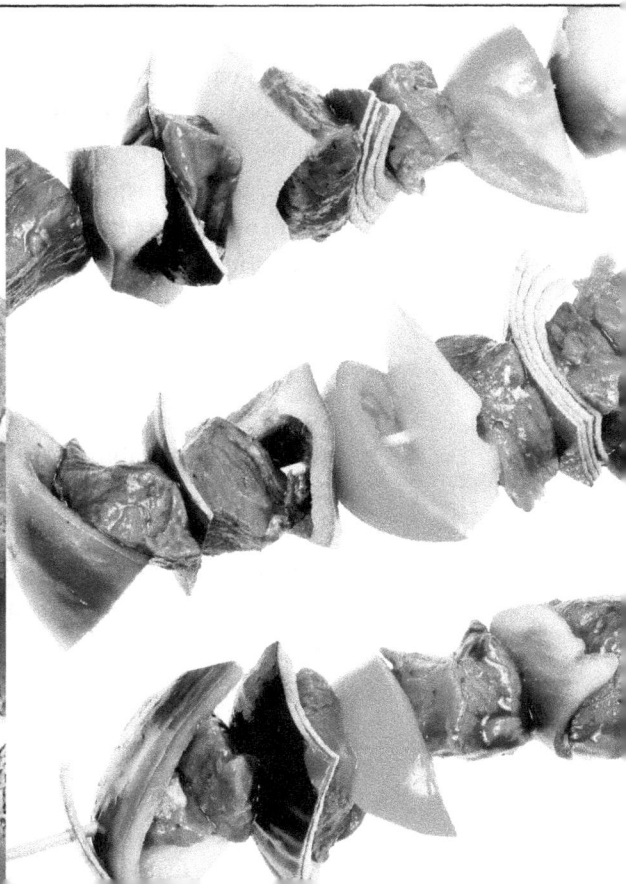

BEEF, LAMB AND VEAL ARE PROMOTED as rich sources of protein, iron, zinc, omega 3 fats and vitamin B12. Advertisements suggesting that brain size and human intelligence depend on eating red meat leave vegetarians and those who choose fish and chicken over red meat insulted by the unfounded implications. There is no doubt that red meat is a good source of these nutrients, but the brain neither knows nor cares where they come from. Kangaroo actually tops the class for most nutrients and also has a low level of fat. Although pork is marketed as a white meat in Australia, researchers include it among the red meats. It has less iron and higher levels of some B complex vitamins than other red meats, but otherwise it fits the general nutritional profile.

Rabbit, hare, goat, poultry (chicken, duck, turkey, quail and other birds) and venison are all low in fat and good sources of protein, iron, zinc and vitamins of the B complex (especially B3, B6 and B12). Wild rabbit, hare, quail and venison have much more iron than beef or lamb.

Medical and scientific studies show no ill effects from eating small amounts of red meat, but researchers are less than enthusiastic about the large portions commonly served in Australia. Meat production also results in environmental problems and an increasing number of people are concerned about the welfare of pigs, poultry and cattle jammed into feedlots. An environmentally friendly diet does not need to exclude animal products – quite the contrary, as animals can be useful ways to enrich soils and recycle some nutrients – but some methods of meat production are less sustainable. The methane that cattle and sheep burp is a potent greenhouse gas, and land used to grow the huge quantites of grain and legumes required for animal fodder could be better used for crops to feed humans. Climate scientists recommend we eat less meat from animals such as sheep and cattle. Sydney University's Centre for Integrated Sustainability Analysis has calculated that halving meat consumption would cut the average Australian's greenhouse gas emissions by almost 25 per cent. Meat producers dispute these figures.

Red meat is a mixed bag – a convenient source of nutrients, and useful in small quantities, but not essential since its nutrients can be supplied by other foods.

126

The 'goodness' in meat

IRON

Iron is used for making haemoglobin, a red pigment in the blood that carries oxygen to cells where it is needed for the production of energy. Meat is a good source of iron, with about 40 per cent of its iron present in a form called haem iron that is well absorbed by the body. Chicken and seafood also contain haem iron. The iron in eggs, legumes, grains and vegetables is called non-haem iron and is less well absorbed than the iron in meat. However, if the body needs more iron, non-haem iron's rate of absorption may increase, often dramatically during pregnancy. A small amount of haem iron in a meal increases the absorption of non-haem iron, so a little meat, fish or chicken helps us absorb more iron from vegetables, legumes or grains.

ZINC

A vital part of brain cells, zinc also assists in growth and repair as required in the skin, liver, pancreas, kidneys, eyes and the prostate gland. Zinc deficiency is rare in Australia, but occurs in some regions of the world where people have very little food and even less food of high nutritional quality. The best sources of zinc – by far – are oysters and mussels, but red meat is also a good source, along with legumes, rolled oats and other cereals, dairy products and some nuts.

PROTEIN

Red meat is high in protein with similar levels to chicken, eggs and seafood. Other sources include legumes, nuts, seeds and grains. The body digests the proteins from any of these foods into amino acids without distinguishing between those that come from meat, milk or muesli. Australians consume more protein than the body requires.

VITAMIN B12

This vitamin is vital for electrical impulses to be transmitted along nerve fibres. It is found only in animal foods – any kind of meat or poultry, seafood, milk, cheese, yoghurt or eggs. Those whose diet contains no animal products need a vitamin B12 supplement or a soy drink with added vitamin B12. Some fruit-eating primates get their vitamin B12 from grubs and insects in the fruit.

Meat from sheep and cattle that are grass fed contains an omega 3 fat called DPA (docosapentaenoic acid). Meat from feedlot cattle (which are fed a high proportion of grain) has virtually no DPA. Without labelling, it is not possible to know whether beef contains this 'good' fat. There has been less research into the benefits of DPA than other omega 3 fats, but it appears to have favourable effects in reducing some undesirable triglyceride fats in the bloodstream. The body can also convert DPA to DHA – the omega 3 fat found in brain tissue. This does not really back the advertising hype about red meat being 'brain food'. Indeed, one study reports that brainier kids are more likely to choose a vegetarian diet!

Hormones in meat

About 40 per cent of beef cattle in Australia are given an ear implant that releases a growth hormone to increase their muscle mass. The meat industry claims this is an advantage because it permits the animal to lay down more muscle in a shorter time. Meat from hormone-implanted cattled is banned in the European Union, where officials have concerns it may have carcinogenic properties. Authorities in Australia and the United States reject such claims. One major Australian supermarket chain, however, is phasing out meat from hormone-implanted cattle.

The 'not so good' in meat

Reports on adverse health effects of red meat first appeared in the 1950s and 60s, when concern centred on saturated fat and its relation-ship with heart disease. Butchers began trimming meat of its selvedge fats and leaner meat became the norm. About this time, meat consump-tion also fell dramatically in Australia and concern dropped, as long as lean meat was chosen.

In 1997, the World Cancer Research Fund (WCRF) examined the evidence and noted that substantial amounts of red meat *probably* increase the risk of colorectal (bowel) cancer. There was also concern that high meat diets could *possibly* increase the risk of cancers of the pan-creas, breast, prostate and kidney. By 2007, concern about breast cancer had fallen, but the WCRF stated unequivocally that the evidence was now *convincing* that red meats and processed meats are a cause of bowel cancer. For red meat and cancers of the oesophagus, lung, pancreas and endometrium, the evidence was rated as *limited*. Examining many more studies in 2011, WCRF now rank the evidence that red and processed meats are causes of bowel cancer as *strong*. And, according to this panel of experts, no amount of processed meat can be confidently shown not to increase risk. (Red meat is defined as beef, lamb, pork or goat and processed meat as any meat preserved by salting, curing, smoking or adding chemical preservatives – for example, ham, bacon, hot dogs and some sausages.)

The marketers of red and processed meats react angrily to the WRCF's reports, ignoring the fact that these experts are careful to state that their recommendations should not be misinterpreted to suggest all red meat should be eliminated.

More problems for the meat industry came from a large study that followed over half a million North Americans over 10 years and analysed the factors associated with 71 250 deaths. After correcting for many possible confounding factors, it found that both men and women who ate the most red meat (averaging 150 g/day) were significantly more likely to have died of heart disease, with cancer deaths not far behind.

A diet low in meat may also benefit bone density – and even the eyes have it! A large study in Melbourne that extended for up to 15 years reported that the 25 per cent of participants who ate red or processed meat 10 or more times a week had an almost 50 per cent increase in their risk of developing age-related macular degeneration. There was no increased risk from chicken, even when it was eaten three or more times a week.

Many studies now point to problems from a high intake of red meat, whereas low intakes of red meat in traditional Mediterranean and Asian dietary patterns tend to be associated with health and longevity. There seems little doubt that we should eat only small amounts of red meat. This is particularly likely to apply to those who follow high-protein diets for weight loss. Contrary to the popular belief that such a diet facilitates weight loss, studies comparing diets with high and

129

more moderate intakes of protein show no difference in results. Dieters may need to find alternative protein-rich foods – or another dietary pattern.

The problems associated with red meat do not apply to chicken and fish. Studies consistently find no adverse effects from chicken, and many find that fish is protective against both cardiovascular disease and cancers.

WHY MEAT MAY BE PROBLEMATIC

The evidence incriminating high consumption of red and processed meats is strongest for bowel cancer, and research has identified several possible mechanisms:

- Suspect compounds called heterocyclic amines or polycyclic aromatic hydro-carbons that are known to be carcinogenic form on meat that is grilled, fried or barbecued. These compounds also form when chicken is cooked in these ways, but chicken is not associated with increased cancer risk, so another inter-action factor must also be involved.
- Carcinogenic N-nitroso compounds form in the bowel when meat is con-sumed.
- Saturated fat in meat may promote insulin resistance or influence faecal bile acids. In countries such as Australia where red meats are often fat-trimmed, the incidence of colorectal cancer still increases with high consumption of meat.
- Haem iron may cause cancerous cells to increase in the wall of the bowel through several possible biochemical mechanisms. Haem iron is a prime sus-pect for colorectal cancer.

Researchers in the United Kingdom have found a correlation between cancer-causing substances in the faecal material of those who eat a lot of red meat compared with vegetarians. Several other studies have impli-cated haem iron in lung cancer and tumours in the colon, and test tube studies show that haem iron increases the invasiveness of human breast cancer cells. Where only small servings of red meat (27 to 42 g per day) are consumed, studies have found no correlation between haem iron intake and colorectal cancer.

The increased risk of cardiovascular disease with diets high in red meat, long thought to be due to its saturated fat content, could also be due to haem iron. Selecting lean red meat will reduce the impact of saturated fat, but will have no effect in reducing possible harm from

130

haem iron. Large quantities of haem iron have also been implicated in inflammation, hypertension and pulmonary disease. Red meat contains about four times as much haem iron as chicken or fish.

It would be a mistake to assume red meat is the sole culprit. Other factors may also play a role – and protective factors in foods such as vegetables, fruits and nuts may be relevant. An Australian scientist from CSIRO has spent years looking for something to protect the colon from the harmful effects of a diet high in red meat. His studies in rats and pigs have shown that a high-amylose maize starch can protect the colon and lower the concentrations of harmful compounds formed from a diet high in red meat.

Adverse environmental effects

The unsustainability of our dietary habits also puts meat under the microscope for its use of water and the greenhouse gases associated with its production. Water is scarce and land for food production is limited in Australia. In some places, animals can graze on areas unsuited to growing crops for human consumption, although their potential to cause serious erosion warrants serious consideration. Using land to grow fertilised, watered pasture for animals does not make ecological sense when the same land can be used to produce food for direct human consumption. Increasing numbers of beef cattle are placed in feedlots, but while this may reduce the amount of land required for the animals themselves, when the resources needed to grow their feed are taken into account, their ecological footprint is large. Over 800 000 hectares of Australian agricultural land are used to produce the 1.5 million tonnes of grain and 815 000 tonnes of roughage that cattle consume annually. Some of this land could be used to produce edible crops for humans.

Animals such as rabbit (a white meat), chicken and other forms of poultry (especially quail) are more efficient converters of food to flesh and have a lower carbon footprint than larger animals. They also do not produce methane. Neither do kangaroos, which also graze on grasses that do not require land clearing and whose large feet do not cause erosion, unlike sheep and cattle. The yield of edible flesh from kangaroos is much lower than from cattle, so any option that allowed meat eaters to switch to kangaroo would need to be coupled with a reduced meat intake.

The take-home message

Health authorities do not recommend that people stop eating red meat entirely, since its nutrients are valuable and there is no evidence that small quantities create problems. The WCRF recommends that consumption of all red meat should not exceed 500 g/week, less than many Australians consume. Recipes in books and magazines commonly include 800–1000 g of red meat for four servings (200–250 g per serve). The Australian Guide to Healthy Eating recommends 3–4 servings (65–100 g cooked weight) a week. The challenge is to convince many of us that a 65 g steak is 'normal'. Cutting out even one beef meal a week (as recommended by the Meatless Mondays initiative) can reduce the production of greenhouse gases, leave more water to be used for growing edible crops and reduce high meat consumption. Filling the dinner plate with vegetables and adding either a small portion of lean meat, or using nuts, seeds or legumes for concentrated protein is also a good recipe for better health.

132

Milk

– which one should you choose?

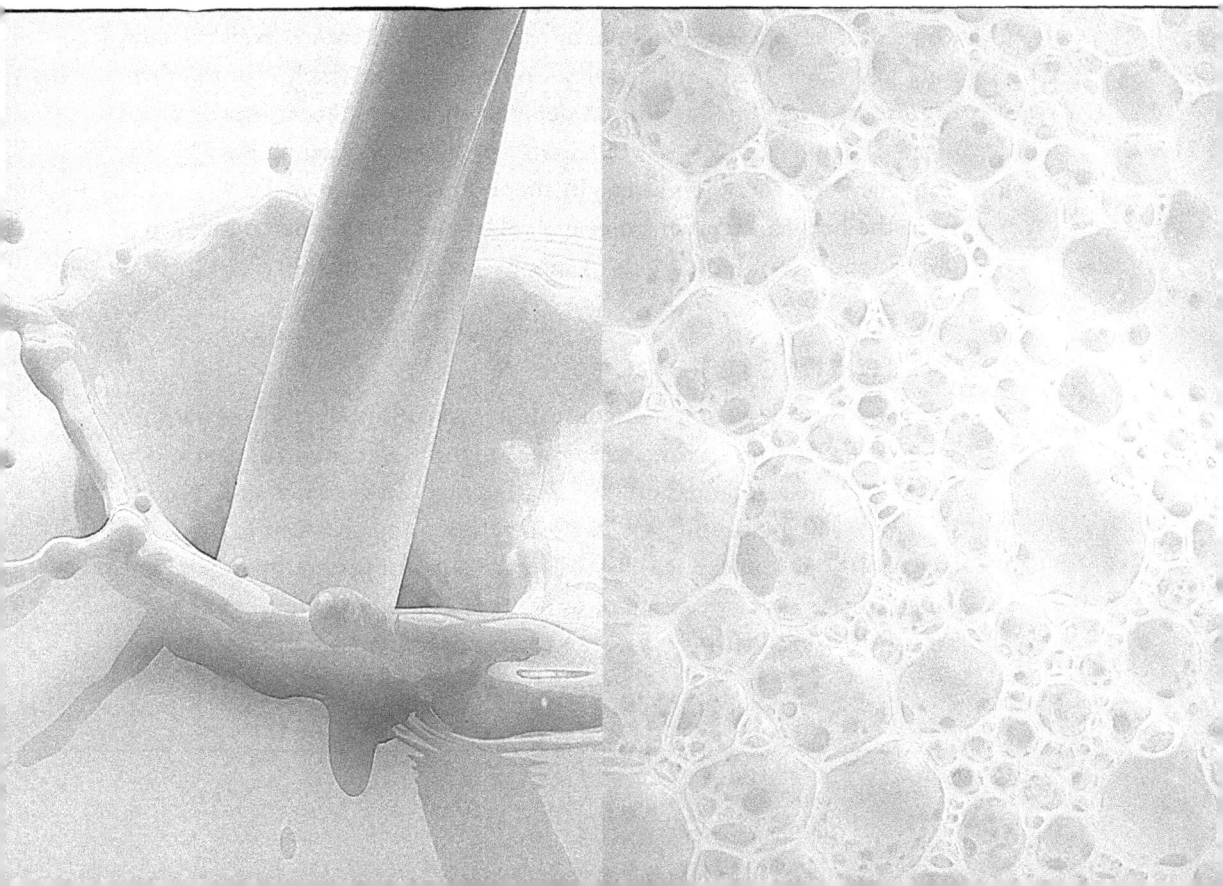

MILK USED TO BE MILK, but these days the dairy cabinet has regular (also called whole or full-cream) milk, reduced-fat (usually reduced to half the usual levels, but other levels are also available), low-fat, skim, a variety of modified milks (some with added skim milk powder to provide extra 'body' and nutrients, others with the usual milk fat replaced with fats from canola oil), milks with added plant sterols, lactose-reduced or lactose-free products, buttermilk, A2 milks and products that are organic or have not been homogenised. On the supermarket shelves you can find powdered milks, evaporated milks with varying levels of fat (plain or flavoured with added sugar), and ultra heat treated (UHT) milks in full cream, reduced fat, skim or modified variations. Most milk sold in Australia is from cows, although milk from goats or sheep is sometimes available. Those who wish to avoid animal products have a choice of milk drinks made from soy, rice or oats. Confused?

Why consume milk?

Milk is an excellent source of protein, calcium, riboflavin (vitamin B2), vitamin B12 (found only in animal products) and iodine, and supplies a range of other minerals and vitamins as well. As it comes from the cow, milk has 3.2–4.5 per cent fat, about 60 per cent of which is in the form of saturated fat. The level of fat depends to a large extent on the breed of cow. Regular milk also contributes pre-formed vitamin A, which is important for young children. In theory, humans can make vitamin A from the beta carotene in fruits and vegetables, but young children may not eat enough of these foods to supply a sufficient quantity.

Lactose intolerance

Humans are unique among mammals in consuming the milk of another species after they are weaned. Mammalian milks all contain a sugar called lactose. Human milk has about 7.2 g lactose/100 g. Cow's milk has 4.8 g lactose/100 g; sheep's milk has 5.1 g/100 g and goat's milk has 4.4 g lactose/100 g. Lactose is digested in the small intestine by an enzyme called lactase. After weaning, most animals stop producing lactase. Many humans also gradually produce less lactase after infancy. Others, however,

134

continue to produce lactase throughout life, giving them the ability to benefit from the nutrients in milk. Continuing to drink milk as a child may prolong the production of lactase, at least in some people. Migrants from countries where milk is not commonly drunk after infancy often find that their children can drink milk without ill effects for many years longer than they could.

When lactase production is reduced, lactose passes to the large intestine where it is fermented by bacteria. This leads to production of gas, which may result in bloating and pain. Diarrhoea may also occur. This condition is called lactose intolerance or lactose maldigestion and is solved by reducing milk consumption. Small quantities of milk do not usually give rise to symptoms, although those who cut out milk from their diet may find that even quite small amounts will produce symptoms. For most people with lactose intolerance, about 12 g of lactose (the amount in 1 cup of milk) spread through the day does not cause symptoms. Regular milk may be better tolerated than reduced-fat milk, as the fat slows the rate of passage through the stomach and into the small intestine.

People with lactose intolerance can still eat cheese, because it contains very little if any lactose, with the possible exception of ricotta, at 2 g lactose/100 g. Yoghurt does not usually cause problems because the bacteria that cause it to thicken partially break down the lactose to its component sugars, glucose and galactose.

Lactose intolerance may occur in children after a bout of gastroenteritis when the inflamed intestine fails to produce enough lactase. Within a couple of weeks after the infection clears, tolerance usually returns.

Those with undiagnosed coeliac disease also have difficulty with lactose, as the lactase enzyme is produced in the area of the intestine that is damaged by gluten. Once gluten is removed from the diet, the intestine recovers and tolerance to lactose returns.

In an extremely rare and life-threatening congenital condition known as primary lactose intolerance, infants are unable to tolerate any lactose, including that in their mother's breast milk, and must from birth be placed on a special diet. This condition should not be confused with the common form of lactose intolerance seen in many populations throughout the world.

Milk allergy

Some children develop skin rashes and other symptoms from drinking cow's milk when the digestive system doesn't break down the protein in cow's milk to its component amino acids. The improperly digested amino acids lead to the body's immune system setting up a reaction. Most allergies to cow's milk disappear by the age of four or five when the digestive system matures sufficiently. Most children who are allergic to cow's milk are also allergic to goat's milk. Children with a true milk allergy, unlike those with lactose intolerance, must avoid all milk products, including ice cream and custard. If a child appears to be allergic to milk, but can tolerate ice cream, the problem does not lie with the milk.

Pasteurisation

All milk sold in Australia is pasteurised, using a process first developed by the Frenchman Louis Pasteur about 150 years ago. Pasteurisation involves heating milk to 72°C for 15 seconds.

Some people oppose pasteurisation because it destroys some of the enzymes in the milk as well as possibly beneficial microbes. Their arguments have a certain validity when it comes to making particular types of cheese, because the flavour of the cheese is different when it is made from raw milk. For milk purchased as a liquid, however, pasteurisation is a highly effective way of destroying the pathogens that can be present in raw milk. These include *Listeria monocytogens*, which can cause abortion, and illness in the frail aged or those who are already ill, *Campylobacter* spp., *Salmonella* spp. and hazardous forms of *Escherichia coli* (*E. coli*), all of which can cause food poisoning and damage the kidneys. Before milk was pasteurised, it was a common cause of many different food-borne illnesses, including tuberculosis, typhoid and Q fever (also known as brucellosis or undulant fever). These serious problems have decreased everywhere pasteurisation of milk has become routine. Pasteurisation does cause some loss of thiamin (vitamin B1) and vitamin C, but milk is a poor source of these, even when unpasteurised. The loss of enzymes is not a valid concern because they are of no importance to humans and are destroyed in the acidic environment of the stomach.

Food authorities in Australia are looking at ways to allow the sale of unpasteurised milk, tested for safety, for those who wish to use it. Some cheeses made from raw milk, certified to be free of harmful pathogens, are already permitted, including Emmental, Gruyère and Sbrinz and Roquefort type cheeses produced under specified conditions.

Homogenisation

If fresh milk is left to stand, the fat (cream) in the milk will rise to the top. This occurs more with cow's milk than the milk from sheep or goats because the fat globules in cow's milk form clusters. Homogenisation is a process whereby the liquid milk is forced through small holes under high pressure to break up any globules and ensure the fat is in small particles which will stay evenly distributed through the milk. The process was invented by another Frenchman, Auguste Gaulin, in 1899. It neither adds nor subtracts anything from the milk and no research supports the belief that homogenisation makes milk fat more harmful to humans. There is no legal requirement for milk to be homogenised, and some organic milk products are sold unhomogenised for those who prefer a layer of cream on top of their milk.

Hormones

Dairy cows in the United States are given a hormone called recombinant bovine somatotropin (rBST) to increase their milk production. Australia and New Zealand ban this hormone – and hopefully this will not change, as hormone-treated cows suffer an increased incidence of mastitis and other health problems.

Which milk?

IN THE BEGINNING

Dietary guidelines recommend that babies are breast-fed solely for six months, then with other foods added and breastfeeding continued for at least 12 months or until appropriate for the particular mother and child. Unmodified cow's milk is not suitable for infants under 12

137

months of age because, compared with breast milk, it has too much protein, phosphorus and sodium (almost four times as much), the wrong balance of fats and B complex vitamins, and not enough carbohydrate and vitamin E. Babies who are not able to be breast-fed need infant formula, although no formula milk can ever match the unique qualities of breast milk. During their second year of life, when children are eating a range of foods and their digestive system has matured, cow's milk can make a major contribution to the nutrients and kilojoules required for growth. For this reason, and also because of its preformed vitamin A, full-cream milk is recommended until two years of age. After that, reduced-fat milk is suitable and may help reduce the amount of saturated fat in the total diet.

REGULAR (FULL-CREAM) MILK

Regular milk sold in Australia must contain a minimum of 3.1 per cent protein and 3.2 per cent fat. The exact quantities vary with the season and the breed of cow. Most milk from the dominant Holstein-Friesian breed has 3.5 per cent protein and 3.5–3.6 per cent fat. Over 60 per cent of milk fat is saturated, a level that can be problematic for cholesterol levels in some people who consume a lot of milk. A cup of milk has 9 g of fat and 5.5 g of saturated fat. When only a small quantity of milk is used, for example added to a cup of tea, changing to reduced-fat milk will have little practical effect.

REDUCED-FAT MILK

Reduced-fat milk has some of the cream removed, leaving 1–2 per cent fat, the exact amount differing with the brand of milk. Removing fat reduces the pre-formed vitamin A level, but this vitamin is easily supplied from beta carotene in fruits and vegetables. The calcium content is at least as high as regular milk and is absorbed as well. Some brands of reduced-fat milk add vitamins A and D.

LOW-FAT MILK

These products vary with the brand, but most contain around 1 per cent fat.

138

SKIM MILK

With virtually no fat content, skim milk tends to have a watery appearance. It has no pre-formed vitamin A but the same calcium content as regular or reduced-fat or low-fat milks.

MODIFIED MILKS

Most modified milks have a reduced fat content and then have skim milk solids added to provide more 'body'. These milks have higher levels of protein, calcium and other nutrients, making them useful for those who wish to maximise the nutrients in milk while minimising the quantity they consume. Their higher lactose content makes them taste sweeter, but means they are less suitable for those with lactose intolerance. Exact concentrations of nutrients vary with different brands, so check the nutrition information panel for specific products. Some have added vitamin D, which is useful for those who cannot expose their skin to sunlight (the usual source of vitamin D). Others boost the calcium content or add various nutrients which are included in the ingredient list.

FAT-MODIFIED MILK

Some milks have all the fat removed and oil added to provide omega 3 or other unsaturated fats. The quantity of fat can be similar to either regular or reduced-fat milks. Research has not shown any problems from the rearrangement of the fats in these products, although nobody really knows whether changing the basic structure of foods in this way could have long-term effects.

PLANT STEROL-MODIFIED MILK

Spreads have had plant sterols added for some years and they are now being added to milk. The sterols prevent cholesterol being absorbed, but they also cause a decrease in the body's ability to absorb protective components from fruit and vegetables. As discussed on page 68, anyone who consumes these products needs to eat an extra daily serving of fruit and vegetables to make up for the losses. There are other ways to reduce cholesterol safely, such as cutting out trans fat and cutting down on saturated fats, especially those found in junk foods. Children and pregnant women should avoid these milks as no tests have been done in these groups.

139

LACTOSE-REDUCED MILK

Most lactose-reduced milk has been treated with lactase, the enzyme that breaks the lactose down to its component sugars, glucose and galactose, and has a sweeter flavour than regular milk.

BUTTERMILK

Years ago, this was the liquid left when cream was whipped into butter. Buttermilk is now made from reduced-fat milk thickened with a bacterial culture similar to those used to produce yoghurt. It has a slightly acidic flavour, is excellent in cooking, and has similar nutrient content to reduced-fat milk.

A2 MILK

Controversy surrounds A2 milk. Normal milk contains a variety of casein and whey proteins. Some of the casein is present in forms called A1 and A2 beta casein, with the proportions varying in the milk from different breeds of cows. The milk of Guernsey and Jersey cows has greater quantities of A2 protein. A2 milk is about twice the price of regular milk and has similar levels of lactose and nutrients to regular milk.

Some people claim that cardiovascular disease and type 1 diabetes are more common in countries where milk has a predominance of A1 beta casein. Since other factors also differ in these countries, most experts need some proof for the superiority of A2 milk. Claims that autism and schizophrenia are caused by A1 beta casein are not backed by evidence at this stage. Further studies by independent scientists are needed.

ULTRA HIGH TEMPERATURE FILTRATION (UHT) MILK

Exposing milk to high temperatures (140°C for 3–5 seconds) destroys bacteria that would normally make the milk go 'off', and allows it to be kept at room temperature for many months. Once opened, the milk must be refrigerated. Most nutrients in UHT milk are unaffected by the treatment, although slight changes in the protein produce a slight caramelisation in the flavour.

EVAPORATED MILK

In making evaporated milk, about 60 per cent of the water is removed from either regular or reduced-fat milk. The nutrients remain in a more concentrated form, with approximately 8.5 per cent protein, 9.5 per cent milk fat and 8.5 per cent lactose. Reduced-fat or skim evaporated milks have approximately 1 per cent fat. Production of evaporated milk changes the protein structure slightly, altering the flavour. A small number of children who are allergic to regular milk can tolerate evaporated milk because of its slightly different protein structure. Once a can of evaporated milk is opened, it must be kept in the fridge.

SOY MILK

Soy milk can be made in the home kitchen by soaking soy beans, draining and grinding them, and then simmering in fresh water for two hours. The drained liquid is soy milk; it provides some protein and nutrients, but little calcium. Most commercially prepared soy milks (or 'soy beverages', as the dairy industry thinks they should be called) are fortified with calcium at the same level as regular milk. A range of vitamins is added, and some brands add vitamin B12, making soy milk a good choice for vegans since B12 is usually found only in animal foods. Check that soy milk has 120 mg calcium/100 mL if it is intended to replace cow's milk. The fat level varies and is usually added from either canola or sunflower oils. Soy milk contains no lactose, but most brands add either sucrose, glucose or malt extract to improve the flavour. Other additives include maltodextrins, sodium bicarbonate and various mineral salts, food acids and gums.

Some internet sites claims that soy milk is harmful. Apart from some soy milk products that contained seaweed from contaminated sources, claims that soy milk is hazardous are unfounded.

RICE MILK

Popular with vegetarians, rice milk is made from rice flour with added canola oil, mineral salts, emulsifiers and other additives. Some brands have added calcium. The protein level is low, so rice milk is not suitable for young children. The carbohydrate is high, with about two-thirds as starch and the rest from added sugar. Some brands add canola oil to add alpha linolenic acid, an omega 3 fat. The longer chain omega 3 fatty acid, DHA, may also be added; this is usually derived from algae rather than fish. The quantity is small, but the added DHA could be significant for those who do not eat seafood. Check for a calcium level of 120 mg/100 mL.

OAT MILK

Made from oat flour with added oil and a sugar such as honey, oat milk is low in protein and fat, but relatively high in sugar. It also contains some dietary fibre. Some brands have added calcium and other nutrients, but the protein content is too low to consider it a suitable replacement for milk for young children. Check that the calcium level is 120 mg/100 mL if oat milk is used as a replacement for cow's milk for older children or adults.

The take-home message

The variety of available milk products makes choice difficult. In general, regular (full-cream) milk is suitable for those under two years of age, with reduced-fat milk recommended as the main type for everyone else.

Nuts

– a healthy harvest

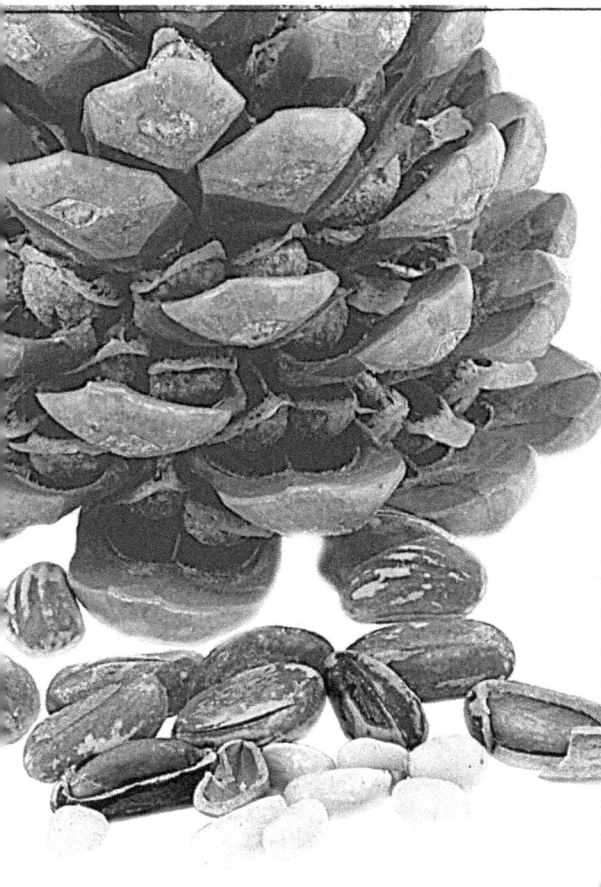

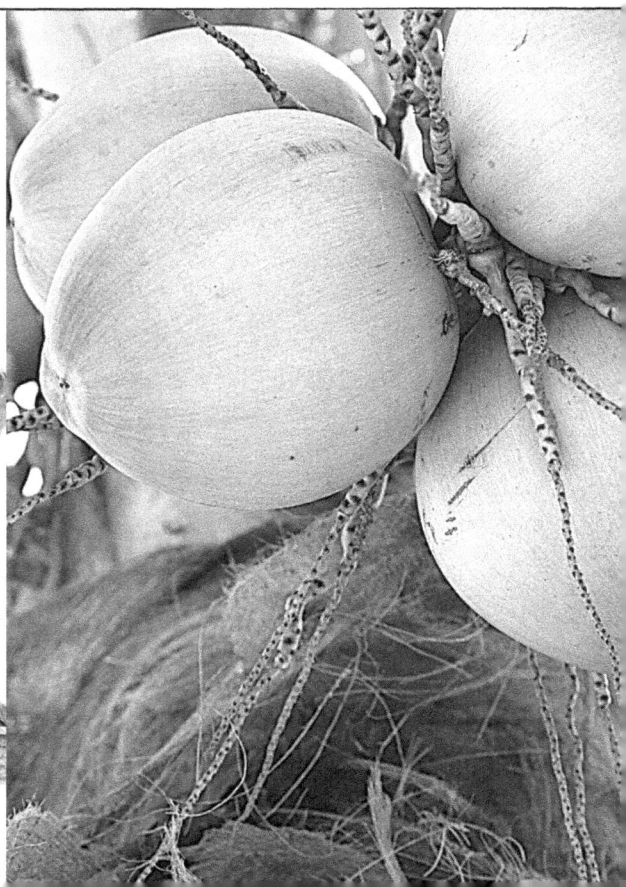

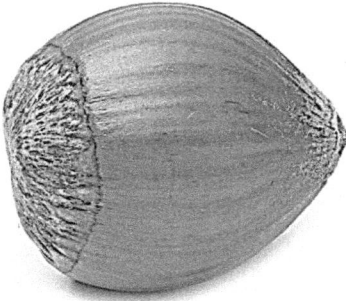

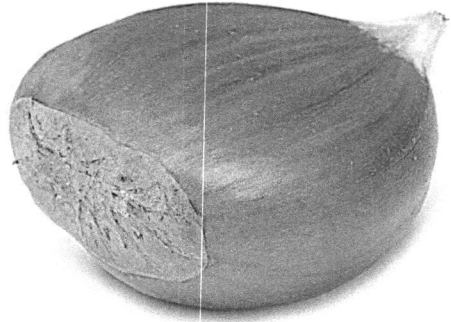

NUTS ARE ONE OF THE ORIGINAL FOODS that our ancestors gathered and it is likely they also played a role in the first human settlements. Excavations in Turkey have uncovered signs of non-migratory groups developing their societies around almond and pistachio trees about 10 000 years ago. Harvesting nuts almost certainly fostered village life and gave rise to the pursuit of agriculture.

Nuts are basic, healthy and delicious foods so why do they give rise to guilt among many people? The reason probably lies in their fat content. Even though the fat in most nuts is the healthy unsaturated kind, many people can't see past the high fat content– although they ignore it when munching on chips, chocolate and cheese. As dozens of studies show the value of discriminating in favour of 'good' fats, nuts are moving to their rightful place as an important part of a healthy diet based on plenty of plant foods.

Not everything we call a nut is technically a nut. Hazelnuts, hickory nuts, chestnuts, walnuts and acorns are true nuts, but in common usage the term 'nut' refers to any hard-walled, edible kernel. Peanuts are really the seeds of a legume, while Brazil nuts, almonds, pistachios and macadamias ('tree nuts') are the seeds of various fruiting trees.

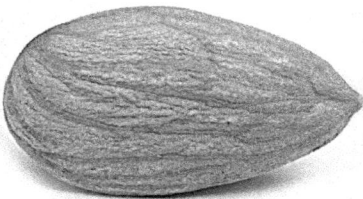

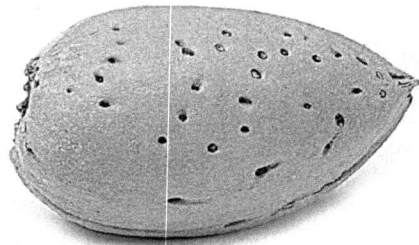

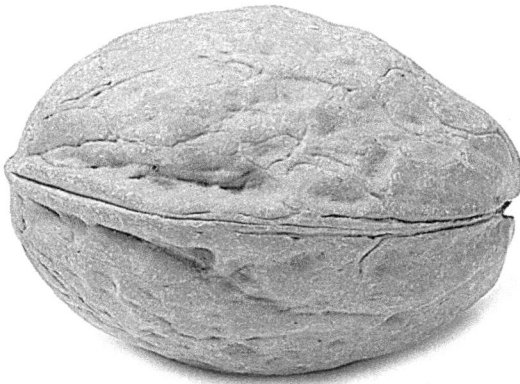

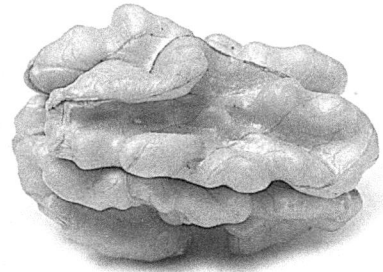

Why they are good for you

As squirrels appreciate, nuts are a concentrated source of nutrients. They contain fat, protein, minerals, vitamins, dietary fibre and a wide range of bioactive substances, including several potent antioxidants. The skin of nuts such as almonds and peanuts is particularly rich in protective antioxidants. At this stage, it is difficult to decide if any single factor in nuts should be lauded, or whether it's the whole neat little package that is so good for us.

FATS

With the exception of chestnuts and bunya nuts, which have almost no fat, most nuts are rich in unsaturated fats. Only coconut fails on this criterion, with a massive 86 per cent of its fat in the form of saturated fat. Almonds, cashews, hazelnuts, macadamias, peanuts, pecans and pistachios are rich in monounsaturated fats – the same healthy kind found in olive oil. Walnuts have more polyunsaturated fats but have a good balance between the omega 3 and omega 6 types. Brazil nuts have roughly equal quantities of mono and polyunsaturated fats. The fats in nuts include some natural sterol compounds

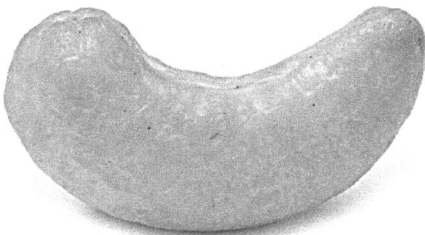

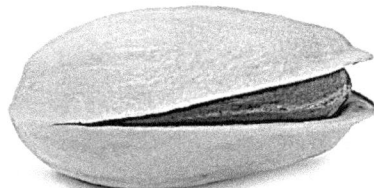

145

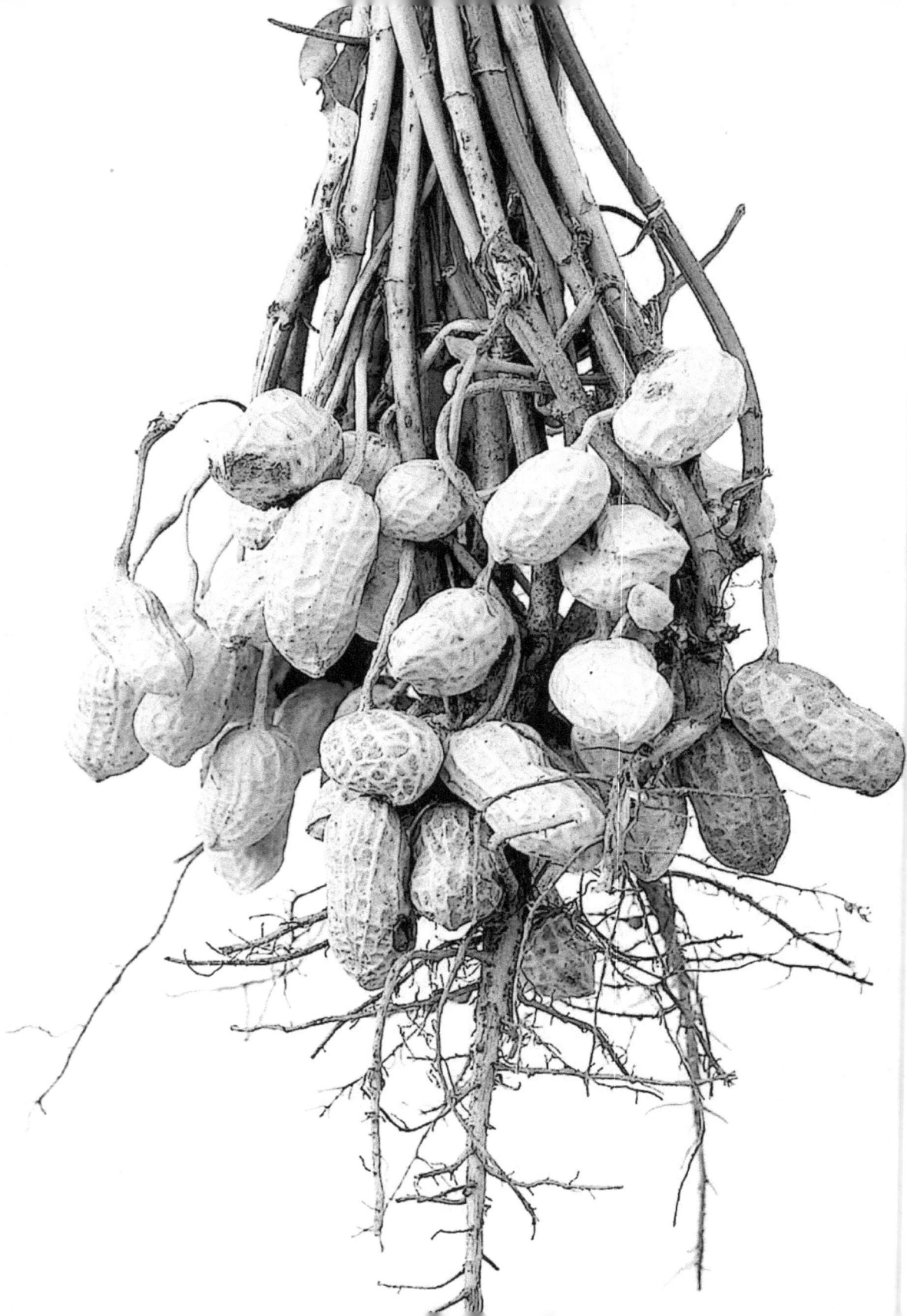

that help prevent cholesterol being absorbed from the intestine and also stop cholesterol already in the arteries from oxidising and forming deposits that will block the blood vessels. These sterols are similar to the compounds extracted from legumes and seeds that are added to expensive sterol-enriched spreads and various dairy products.

PROTEIN

The protein content of nuts ranges from a low 3 per cent in fresh coconut to about 25 per cent in peanuts. Proteins are made up of amino acids, one of which, arginine, is possibly the most exciting component of nut protein. Arginine is converted in the body to a compound that helps blood vessels relax and cardiologists believe it may explain the protection nuts provide against heart disease. Arginine may also help reduce some inflammatory compounds that are risk factors for diabetes and cardiovascular disease.

VITAMINS

Nuts are uniformly high in vitamins, especially the B complex vitamins folate and vitamin B6, with peanuts pipping the rest for their high content of niacin (vitamin B3). Nuts are also rich sources of several forms of vitamin E. Vitamin E consists of eight different compounds called tocopherols and tocotrienols. Some, such as gamma tocopherol, found in high quantity in pistachios, walnuts, pecans and pine nuts, have been largely ignored until recently, but are turning out to have an important protective effect for good health. Hazelnuts, almonds, pine nuts, and peanuts are rich in alpha tocopherol, an important antioxidant that is well absorbed by the body.

MINERALS

The minerals in nuts are no less impressive and emphasise the value to be gained eating a variety of nuts. For example, almonds are especially high in calcium, Brazil nuts are the richest known source of selenium, pine nuts have particularly high levels of iron and zinc, pistachios are rich in potassium, cashews are tops for copper and macadamias dominate the nut class for manganese.

147

GADO GADO SALAD

There's no way this hearty salad could be called rabbit food!

PEANUT SAUCE

2 teaspoons sesame oil
1 onion, finely chopped
1 clove garlic, crushed
1 teaspoon dried shrimp paste
140 g tomato paste, no added salt
½ cup crushed peanuts
2 tablespoons peanut butter
¾ cup coconut milk (or water, to reduce saturated fat)
1 tablespoon lime juice
2 teaspoons salt-reduced soy sauce

SALAD

Hardboiled eggs, sliced steamed potatoes, thin wedges of Chinese cabbage, carrot sticks, strips of red capsicum, lightly steamed green beans, asparagus and snow peas

1. Heat oil in a small saucepan and sauté onion and garlic over a gentle heat for 3 minutes. Add shrimp paste, tomato paste, peanuts, peanut butter and coconut milk and cook, stirring, for 5 minutes. Add lime juice and soy sauce.

2. On a platter, arrange an attractive selection of vegetables. Top with sliced hardboiled eggs and drizzle the peanut sauce over the salad.

The peanut sauce is also ideal to serve with skewers of grilled chicken or any barbecued skewered vegetables. Try button mushrooms, chunks of zucchini and squares of red capsicum.

Blend chick peas with garlic, lemon juice, tahini and enough of the cooking water or canned liquid to form a thick paste.

148

All nuts are excellent sources of dietary fibre, including both soluble and insoluble types.

Eat nuts for your health

Initially, researchers were interested in nuts because of their important role in Mediterranean diets. More than 20 studies from around the world have now reported positive health benefits from specific kinds of nuts. These trials have shown that nuts decrease total and LDL ('bad') cholesterol levels in the blood, presumably because of their high content of unsaturated fats. Nuts also lead to lower concentrations of inflammatory compounds related to the health of blood vessels.

Studies also show that several compounds in tree nuts and peanuts may protect against gallstone disease in both men and women.

Nuts and weight gain

Nuts are high in kilojoules and so have always been tagged as fattening. The evidence from many studies, however, does not confirm this assumption. This does not mean that kilojoules don't count – they do. But other factors obviously come into play, since many studies show an inverse relationship between frequency of nut consumption and body fat. Those who consume nuts regularly are less likely to be obese and have a much lower risk of type 2 diabetes. It appears that nuts help to regulate the appetite. Because they are filling, those who eat some nuts are less likely to consume an excess of other foods.

In many studies where participants have been given 30–50 g of nuts a day, there has been no weight gain. In some trials where subjects were simply asked to eat nuts each day, weight loss has occurred. There is also some evidence that nuts decrease the absorption of fats, with some trials showing higher levels of fat in the stools after consuming nuts.

NUTTY IDEAS

Nuts are often considered only as a snack food, but they deserve to be incorporated into meals.

The flavour of nuts is much better if you toast them lightly on a dry frying pan before use. Use only a moderate heat and watch carefully as they burn easily.

Sprinkle toasted slivered almonds over steamed green beans or asparagus – the vegetables taste better and you get a nutrient boost.

Toast a few chopped walnuts. Cook sliced onions and garlic in a little olive oil, add a bunch of washed shredded English spinach and combine with cooked drained pasta. Top with walnuts.

Make a pesto with pine nuts and either basil or parsley. Or use macadamia nuts, almonds or walnuts in place of pine nuts. Serve with steamed potatoes, spread on toast and top with tomatoes, add a dollop to soups or serve with pasta or grilled fish.

Scatter a few toasted pecans or pistachios over the top of a salad of peeled sliced oranges and pink grapefruit and serve for breakfast, at lunchtime or as a dessert.

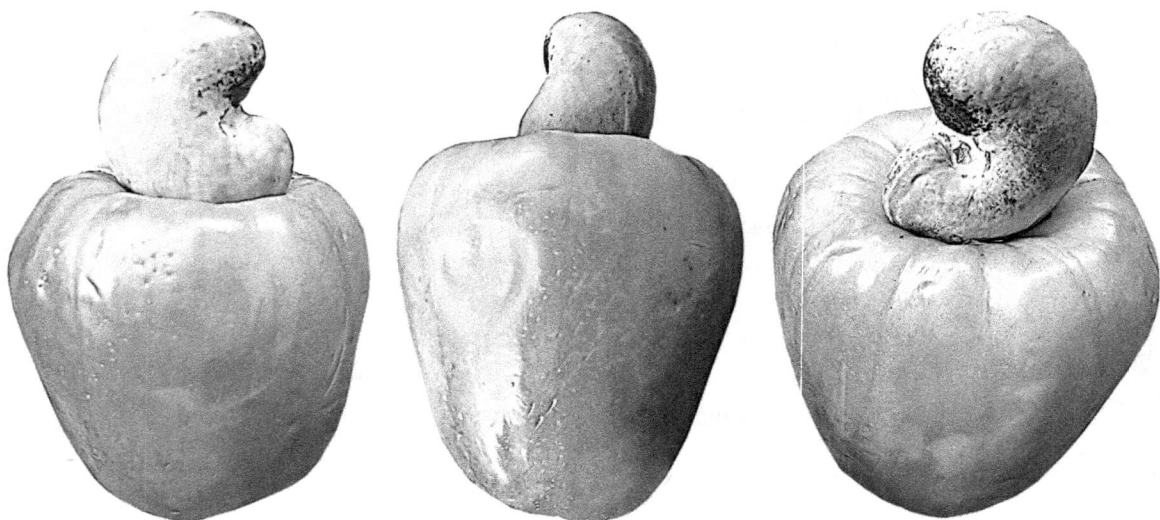

CASHEWS – THE FRUIT AS WELL AS THE NUT IS EDIBLE

Nut allergies

Peanuts and tree nuts feature among the eight most common sources of allergens that cause a range of allergic symptoms. (Note that food *intolerances*, as opposed to *allergies*, do not involve the body's immune system and can come and go at any age or stage of life.) A small, but increasing number of children suffer an allergic reaction to tree nuts or peanuts and a few react to both. Whereas most children 'grow out' of their food allergies as their digestive systems mature, about 80 per cent of children with peanut allergy retain it for life. Peanut allergy can be severe, leading to anaphylaxis, a multi-system reaction which is potentially fatal. This is rare, fortunately – most cases of peanut allergy result in symptoms such as skin rashes or hives. Unfortunately, we have no way of knowing if a child with peanut allergy might have an anaphylactic reaction so any peanut allergy must be taken seriously.

It's worth noting that it's extremely rare for an anaphylactic reaction to occur unless the child actually consumes peanuts. In one study reported in the *Journal of Allergy and Clinical Immunology*,* when 30 peanut-allergic children were exposed to peanut butter, either on their skin for 1 minute, or on a large surface area held 30 cm from their faces for 10 minutes, one-third of the children with peanut butter on their skin had a reaction. In three children, the skin appeared red, five felt itchy (but had no obvious signs of a rash) and two developed a weal where the peanut butter had been. None had a serious reaction and none of the 30 children had any reaction from being close to peanut butter. The researchers reported that casual exposure to peanut butter was unlikely to lead to any significant allergic reactions, although they noted this could not be generalised to longer or larger exposure or to contact with peanut in forms such as peanut flour and roasted peanuts.

All children with a serious allergy to peanuts or any other food need to have access to an EpiPen containing a ready dose of adrenalin. A study at the Children's Hospital at Westmead, Sydney,** reported that children with an allergic reaction to seafood were five times more likely to suffer an anaphylactic reaction than those allergic to peanuts.

* Steven J Simonte et al, 'Relevance of casual contact with peanut butter in children', *Journal of Allergy and Clinical Immunology*, 2003;112(1): 180–82.
** David Brill, 'Seafood a major anaphylaxis trigger in kids', *Annals of Allergy, Asthma and Immunology*, 2011; 106: 494–501.

DID YOU KNOW?

- Hazelnuts are called filberts in some parts of the world.
- Hawaii is the world's largest producer of macadamia nuts, but they are native to Australia.
- Walnuts originated in Persia (now Iran), as did pistachios, but both are widely used in Indian cuisine as well.
- Pecans are native to North and South America.
- Bunya nuts from the Australian bunya pine have a dryish texture a bit like chestnuts. Don't sit under a bunya tree because a single cone (weighing up to 7 kg) may fall unexpectedly! Potentially a killer nut …
- The saturated fats in coconut are not all 'bad', but neither are they all 'good' as some websites proclaim. Some of the fatty acids, the short-chain type, do not have any adverse effects on blood cholesterol, but coconut also contains saturated fatty acids that do have the potential to raise blood cholesterol.
- Nuts are an environmentally friendly food; nut trees store carbon, require little fertiliser and produce crops for many years.

Oils
– which one?

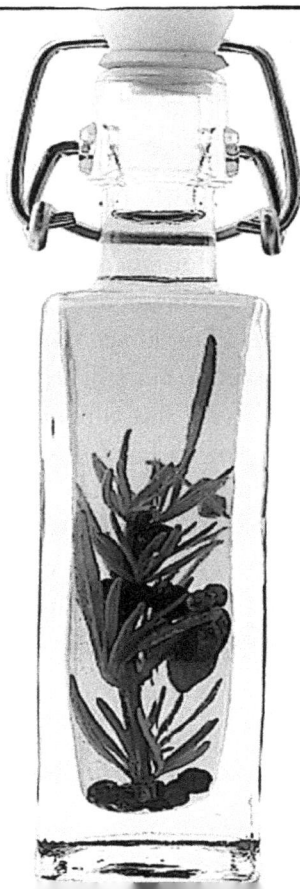

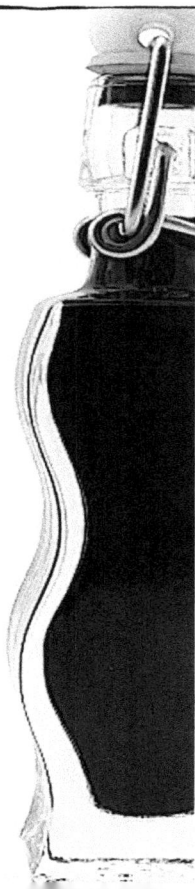

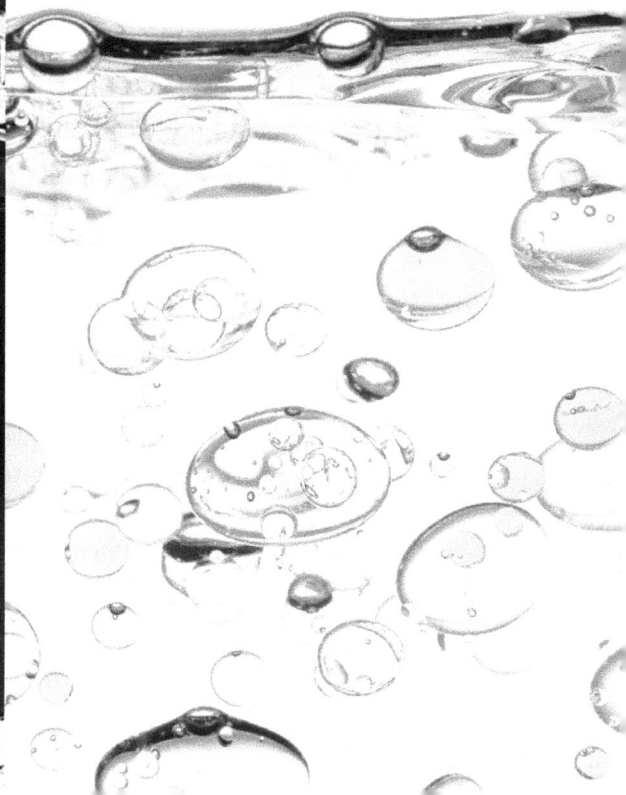

UNTIL THE 1960s, most Australian kitchens had a pot for dripping collected from roasting beef and another for lard from bacon and pork. Dripping was used for roasting and frying; lard was used for making crisp pastry. Liquid oils were rarely used, except by migrants from Mediterranean countries who bought and used their beloved olive oil. At that time, most Anglo-Saxons rejected olive oil as 'greasy', although they may have kept a small bottle (bought at a pharmacy, and often so ancient it was rancid) in the bathroom cupboard for external use.

By the 1970s, dripping and lard had all but disappeared and most people had turned to vegetable oils for cooking. Initially, the most popular oils were corn (also called maize), safflower, sunflower, soybean or a mixed blend of any of these oils. Sesame oil is also a polyunsaturated oil, used mainly in Asian cuisines, and grape seed oil became popular a little later. Monounsaturated oils, mainly olive, canola and peanut are also popular, with olive oil now the dominant domestic oil in Australia, followed by canola. High-end restaurants often cook with peanut or olive oil, but most commercial fast-food outlets use either a mixture of oils containing canola, cottonseed, palm or sunflower oils or a 'solid' oil containing high levels of trans fat from partially hydrogenated vegetable oils.

Are they good for you?

Any liquid oil is nutritionally superior to lard which in turn is better than dripping which is better than the 'solid' vegetable oil often used in commercial frying. Liquid oils are best because they contain mainly unsaturated fats and no trans fat. Dripping has the disadvantage that 55 per cent of its fat is saturated. Lard is slightly better but still has 41 per cent saturated fat. The 'solid' commercial frying fats contain either a high level of saturated fat or up to 50 per cent trans fat – the worst kind of fat.

The fats in liquid oils actually contain a mixture of polyunsaturated, monounsaturated and saturated fatty acids, but are usually classified by the dominant type. For example, corn, safflower, sunflower, soybean, grape seed and sesame oils are largely polyunsaturated, although they contain some monounsaturated and saturated fat. The dominant fatty acids in olive, canola, rice bran, mustard seed, macadamia and peanut oils are monounsaturated. The tropical palm, palm kernel and coconut oils used in biscuits, crackers, crisps, cakes and fried or frozen foods are high in saturated fat.

The kind of polyunsaturated fats we consume is the subject of much debate among scientists. There are two types designated according to their chemical structure as omega 3s or omega 6s. Most polyunsaturated oils contain omega 6 fatty acids. Omega 3 polyunsaturated fats are found in fish and seafood, and also in linseeds, canola and walnuts. Many researchers argue that the addition of polyunsaturated oils and margarines to our diet has unbalanced the desirable ratio between the two classes of polyunsaturated fatty acids and this may alter the body's production of chemicals that control inflammatory reactions and blood pressure. Unusually large quantities of omega 6 fats can also reduce 'good' HDL cholesterol in the blood, although studies show a lower incidence of heart disease in those who consume more polyunsaturated fats. Some trials have also shown that the ratio of omega 6 to omega 3 fatty acids correlates with the incidence of certain cancers.

Few human populations ever consumed large quantities of omega 6 fats until processors found a way to extract oils from seeds and grains. Using oils such as olive oil, which has been around for at least 6000 years, or canola, macadamia or peanut oil gets around the issue because these oils are low in polyunsaturated fat. Their major fat, oleic acid, is an omega 9 fatty acid.

Researchers continue to debate the merits of mono and polyunsaturated oils. The most persuasive evidence favours monounsaturated oils because of their lower tendency to oxidise, both in the frying pan and in the body. Other components in oils and the way they are processed are also important. Processing with heat or chemical solvents can destroy many protective plant compounds. This gives extra virgin olive oil a double advantage, since it is processed without heat or chemical solvents and contains more than 30 potentially valuable compounds. Studies show some of these are potent antioxidants and others have specific properties that can help reduce high blood pressure. These extra factors in olive oil may help explain the lower incidence of many types of cancer in Mediterranean populations. Or it may be that olive oil simply makes vegetables more enjoyable and much more likely to be eaten.

Oils in processed foods

Once extracted, liquid vegetable oils go 'off' easily, creating problems for use incommercial frying or as ingredients in processed foods. To avoid problems with unsaturated liquid oils, manufacturers use the process of hydrogenation to convert some of the unsaturated fatty acids into saturated fats which have a longer shelf life and melt at a higher temperature. The resulting 'solid' oil produces crisper fried and baked foods. When food companies were required to list saturated fat in the nutrition information panel on their food labels, they began to produce partially hydrogenated oils. This process produces a trans fat called elaidic acid, technically an 'unsaturated' fat that does not need to be listed on labels, and so was seen as more appealing to health-conscious shoppers.

Elaidic acid has no redeeming features. It increases 'bad' LDL cholesterol, decreases 'good' HDL cholesterol and has adverse effects on several other types of fat that create risk for coronary heart disease and Alzheimer's disease. Normal fat-splitting enzymes in the intestine take longer to break down trans fat, which may contribute to its ill effects. Experts agree that there is no safe level of this particular trans fat. Other types of trans fats occur naturally in the milk and meat of ruminant animals. The type in milk, conjugated linoleic acid (CLA) may be beneficial, although results from different studies vary and research continues.

It's now a mistake to think saturated fats are synonymous with animal fats when over 40 per cent of Australians' saturated fat intake now comes from vegetable oils that have been changed through processing.

New oils

Through genetic modification and traditional plant breeding methods, scientists are developing oilseeds with lower levels of omega 6 polyunsaturated fatty acids and more monounsaturates.

Canola oil was originally produced from rapeseeds, and contained a fat called erucic acid which damages the liver and made it a hazardous product until selective breeding eliminated the erucic acid. Genetic modification has resulted in the development of a new variety of canola that is resistant to particular herbicides which many people are opposed to on the grounds that the safety tests that were done before its release were inadequate. There are also problems keeping the GM canola separate from regular canola.

Because canola oil contains some omega 3 fatty acids, it goes rancid easily, and much of it is therefore partially hydrogenated, producing a commercial frying fat high in trans fat. To counter this and produce a cheap oil that is useful in confectionery, biscuits and pastry products, another variety is being genetically modified to have high levels of saturated fatty acids. At this stage, inadequate labelling regulations make it difficult to distinguish between different types of canola oil. The only choice for those wanting non-GM canola oil low in saturated fat is to buy liquid canola oil certified as organic.

Choosing an oil

If the aim is just to reduce total and 'bad' LDL blood cholesterol, polyunsaturated oils do the job most efficiently, although for elderly people, some studies show that omega 6 fats from these oils may contribute to depression, associated with mild cognitive impairment. Any monounsaturated oil will also lower LDL if used in place of saturated fats, and this benefit is unaffected by the degree of refining. However, studies show that the higher levels of antioxidants in extra virgin olive oil have the added benefit of protecting cholesterol in the arteries gainst harmful oxidation. Polyphenolic components in extra virgin olive oil can also reduce high blood pressure whereas polyunsaturated oils do not. Other studies show a range of benefits, with extra virgin olive oil helping to prevent blood cells clumping together, especially after a rich meal.

There is some confusion about the term 'extra virgin'. Modern machinery grinds up the whole olive and centrifuges the resultant paste to extract the oil in a single operation. This produces a superior oil which has little time to deteriorate, as used to happen with older techniques whereby the olives were pressed between straw mats that inevitably held oxidised material. Terms such as 'first cold pressing' are no

157

longer relevant. To be classified as extra virgin, olive oil is tested for free fatty acids (a sign of deterioration) and must meet other criteria for flavour and an absence of defects. Extra virgin olive oil shows the intricate relationship between flavour and nutritional value since many of the components that contribute to its unique fruity flavour are also those that have extra health benefits. For health and taste, extra virgin olive oil has a clear edge over other oils.

Olive oil that doesn't meet the strict criteria for classification as 'extra virgin' can be set aside as 'virgin' oil or further refined to form 'light' olive oil. The 'light' refers to its lack of colour (and flavour), not its fat content, which is the same as for any other oil. A blend of virgin olive oil and light oil was previously called 'pure' olive oil, but is now officially labelled as 'olive oil'. The 'cake' remaining after the extraction process contains small amounts of oil and can be used as fuel (useful to heat factories since olives are harvested in winter), or treated with solvents to extract the last remnants, which are sold cheaply as pomace oil.

Did you know?

- Vegetable oils can be commercially processed to form trans fats but this reaction cannot be duplicated in the home kitchen.
- Polyunsaturated fats deteriorate when heated, forming some oxidised compounds that could disrupt cell membranes – but do not turn into saturated fat as is sometimes alleged. Discard any leftover polyunsaturated oil used for deep frying, preferably by leaving it at a collection point for recycling.
- Extra virgin olive oil retains more of its unique components when used as a dressing, but it can also be heated without ill effect, as the large number of different antioxidants prevents its fats from oxidising. As long as it is strained to remove 'bits' of food, olive oil can be re-used for frying at least 10 times.
- Flaxseed (also called linseed) oil is rich in omega 3 polyunsaturated fat – so much so that it oxidises readily. It needs to be pressed and kept cold at all stages of its short life – or preferably used on cricket bats, where its rapid oxidation is an asset. Better to eat the seeds themselves since their protective coating prevents rapid oxidation of the fats inside.
- All oils are 100 per cent fat and all have the same high kilojoule count – 3700 kJ/100 g.

158

Organically
grown foods

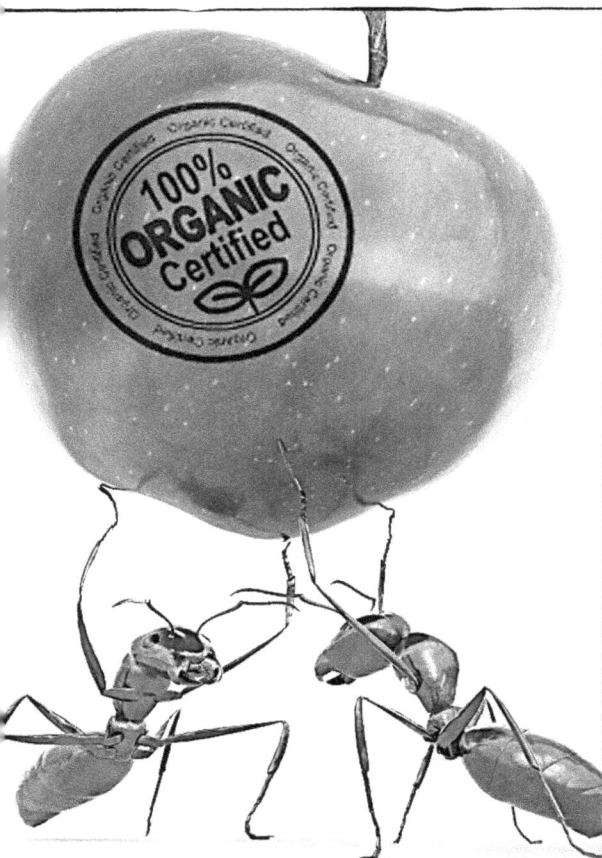

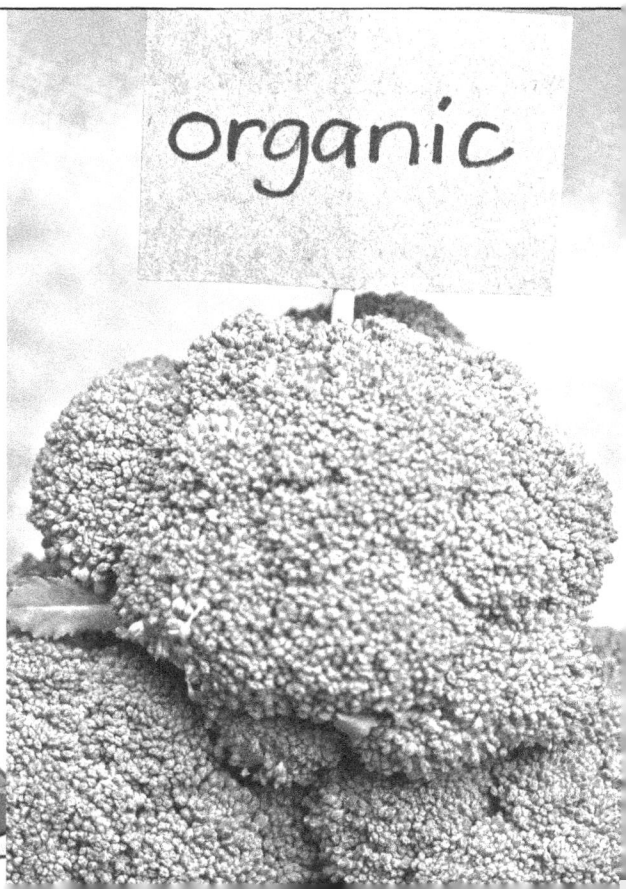

100%
ORGANIC
Certified

organic

GROWERS AND SELLERS OF ORGANIC FOODS are disappointed when some nutritionists don't share their enthusiasm. The media inevitably picks up on any disagreements, as happened with a recent (2009) report commissioned by the UK Food Standards Agency which concluded that organic foods do not contain significantly higher quantities of nutrients than foods produced from conventional agriculture. Organic food groups felt cheated and wondered how the authors could have reached such a conclusion.

In fact, the British group had not done any fresh testing, having merely collated and summarised previous reports. A study was included only if it fitted scientific control principles, and compared conventional and organic plant and animal products produced under similar conditions. This resulted in the majority of studies on organic foods being rejected because there was no exact control. Only nutrients (mostly vitamins, minerals and fats) were compared, with no examination of residual levels of pesticides, fungicides or herbicides. Nor did the report look at flavour or issues connected with sustainability (such as fertiliser use), although it did acknowledge that these issues could be important. These omissions received much less publicity than the comparisons of minerals and vitamins.

Nutrient levels in samples of any crop vary. One cauliflower is not going to have levels of nutrients identical to those in another cauliflower in the same field, let alone one grown earlier or later in the season or in different climatic conditions. So it was not surprising that the nutrient levels in both conventional and organic crops fitted within the general spread of expected results.

A few studies have reported the presence of more natural plant compounds (phytonutrients) in organic crops. These may have potential anti-cancer benefits, but not enough research has yet been done to make a meaningful comparison between plant products within a category or with different production methods.

160

Vitamins and minerals

Very little, if any, difference in vitamin and mineral content has been found in most studies of conventionally and organically grown foods. Where differences do occur, they are slight and largely irrelevant. In the British summary of comparable analyses, the conventional crops had slightly higher levels of nitrogen, the organic crops had a little more magnesium, zinc and phosphorus, but none of these small differences has much practical effect. To put this into perspective, if, say, an organically grown orange has 100 mg vitamin C and a conventionally grown one of the same size has only 90 mg, the difference has little relevance, considering that oranges do not all come in the same size and our need for vitamin C ranges from about 40 to 60 mg/day. Slight differences in levels of vitamins and minerals do not provide a valid reason to choose organic produce.

Residues

There is plenty of evidence that certified organic produce has low chemical residue levels. Australian foods in general have commendably low levels of residues, but less is always better, so this aspect falls in favour of organic produce.

Animal welfare

If you don't like battery-caged hens, cattle kept in feedlots, pigs in small crates, antibiotics used as growth promotants and beef cattle being given extra hormones, organic is the only choice.

Genetic modification (GM) – the bottom line

There is a lack of independent long-term safety studies on GM foods. With more than 10 years of use in the United States, it is obvious that GM crops don't kill people. Some claim they are the reason for the increasing incidence of allergies, but without labelling and testing, it is not possible to agree with or deny such allegations. In Australia, foods

161

containing GM proteins must be labelled, but there is no requirement to label GM oils (such as canola) or sugars. If you prefer to avoid GM ingredients, choose organic foods.

Flavour

Organic farmers often grow a wider variety of products and their generally smaller farms mean that products can be picked at the optimal stage for flavour. Flavour benefits have been confirmed by blind taste tests for some foods.

Carbon footprint

Organic produce can have a lower carbon footprint than conventional produce. Some have similar (or greater) yields to conventional produce and may have a lower carbon footprint because they are grown without conventional fertilisers, herbicides and pesticides. For others the yields are equivocal. Free-range eggs and meat products will usually provide less food per hectare because the animals are given more space. The lower yield will make the products more expensive, but that can be a boon for health if it reduces consumption of products such as red meat (which will then have a lower carbon footprint). Imported organic foods such as confectionery (which no one really needs) may have a high carbon footprint due to their long journey. The carbon footprint for organic foods varies for different products and no overall conclusion can be drawn for their advantages or disadvantages in this criterion. This may change with the increasing scarcity of the phosphate rock required for making superphosphate fertilisers for the conventional products.

Cost

Organic production methods are more labour intensive, which makes some organic produce more expensive than conventionally produced crops. Overall, prices are generally falling as organic products move into major supermarkets. Organic home or community vegetable gardens can be cost-saving alternatives.

162

Certification

In the past, a few unscrupulous non-organic growers claimed organic status for imperfect or blemished produce that did not meet the public's/supermarket chains' standards of appearance. Australia now has a National Standard (administered by the Australian Quarantine Inspection Service) to ensure organic products are genuine. Check for a symbol from one of the following seven organisations:

- National Association for Sustainable Agriculture (NASAA)
- Australian Certified Organic
- Organic Growers of Australia (OGA)
- Organic Food Chain (OFC)
- Safe Food Queensland
- Tasmanian Organic-Dynamic Producers (TOP)
- Bio-dynamic Research Institute (BDRI)

Fit for the future

The last word on this subject should go to Swiss researchers, who have found that soils on farms managed by organic principles are much healthier and house a larger and more diverse community of organisms. That may become the most important consideration in the organic debate and a good reason to choose organic foods.

Salt
– how much is too much?

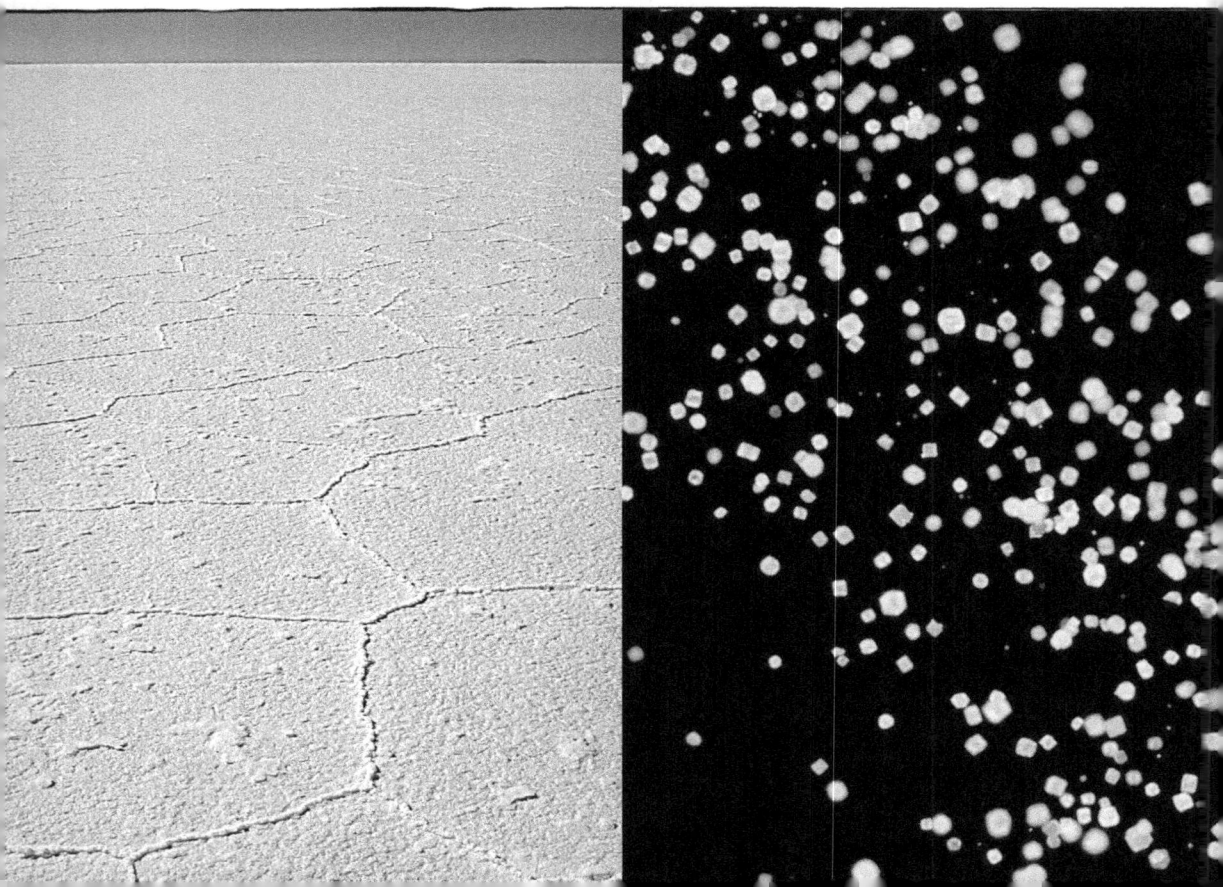

THERE IS NO SHORTAGE OF RESEARCH papers showing the harmful effects of too much sodium from salt. A 2009 analysis published in the *British Medical Journal* examined 13 studies that had followed more than 170 000 people for up to 19 years and found that the more salt they consumed, the greater their risk of stroke and heart disease.* Yet a recent study that followed 3700 Europeans for eight years reported that those who consumed the most salt had *fewer* deaths from heart disease than those who ate less salt.** Critics of this study noted, however, that a higher intake of salt did increase systolic blood pressure (the upper figure in a typical blood pressure measurement that indicates how hard the heart has to work to pump blood around the body). The World Health Organization recently noted that half of all heart attacks and over 60 per cent of strokes are due to high blood pressure.

How much salt do we need?

Salt is sodium chloride. Our bodies don't actually need salt as such, although we do need some sodium to help balance the fluid inside our cells and in the spaces between them. Sodium makes up 40 per cent of salt but it also exists quite naturally in all types of seafood, eggs, meat, dairy products and some vegetables. If you follow a strict vegan diet, you probably need to include foods with added salt (bread perhaps), but omnivores can easily meet their sodium needs without extra salt or salted foods.

Too much sodium causes extra fluid to be retained by the body and this in turn leads to the arteries losing their elasticity – 'hardening of the arteries'. This means the heart has to work harder and blood pressure rises.

The evidence against salt began to accumulate with observations of traditional societies such as the Bushmen of the Kalahari, the Yanomama

---

*   Pasquale Strazzullo et al, 'Salt intake, stroke, and cardiovascular disease: Meta-analysis of prospective studies', *British Medical Journal*, 2009; 339:b4567.

** Katarzyna Stolarz-Skrzypek et al, 'Fatal and nonfatal outcomes, incidence of hypertension, and blood pressure changes in relation to urinary sodium excretion', *Journal of the American Medical Association*, 2011; 305(17): 1777–85.

Indians of Brazil, and various tribes in New Guinea and Australia that had not been exposed to modern processed foods with their high salt content. These groups showed no increase in blood pressure with age, and high blood pressure (hypertension) was virtually unknown. It's not rocket science to note that their lifestyle was also different in other ways. A high intake of vegetables and fruit meant these groups consumed more potassium, a nutrient that helps reduce blood pressure. They were also lean because their total kilojoule intake was balanced with their physical activity. Could it be that some people were genetically programmed to resist hypertension, scientists wondered. The notion was disproved when these groups were introduced to processed foods, and their members experienced the same rise in blood pressure as occurs in the developed world.

Adults need 460–920 mg sodium/day. The upper limit set for safe consumption is 2300 mg/day. Translating this into teaspoons of salt is invalid, because it ignores the sodium present naturally in foods. When people eat mainly fresh foods cooked without salt, and a piece of cheese or a couple of slices of bread, daily sodium intake will be about 1200 mg. Adding processed foods can raise that at least 5-fold to levels that are potentially hazardous if consumed regularly.

Salted foods

About 80 per cent of the salt we consume is already in the foods we buy. Some foods taste obviously salty (for example soy and many other sauces, salted nuts and packet soups) but in others a combination of salt and sugar disguises the amount of salt. Cornflakes generally contain more salt than potato crisps, but the sugar in the cornflakes deceives the tastebuds so they don't taste salty. Without added sugar or salt, cornflakes would have very little taste; even with these additives it is difficult to detect the flavour of corn.

Salt is added to bread for flavour, to help control the action of yeast and to retain moisture. (Unsalted bread dries out rapidly.) Cheeses also have added salt, which acts as a preservative, as it does in salted meats such as ham, bacon and salami. Marinaded meats, poultry and seafood have high levels of salt (and also sugar). Most sauces are high in salt, especially soy, fish and oyster sauces. Packet and canned soups have so little of any real ingredient that they rely on salt for flavour. Crackers and savoury snack foods are also high salt items. Salt is automatically added to foods such as ice creams, desserts and cakes, although there is no technical or taste reason for doing so.

The salt added to processed foods, fast foods and restaurant meals contributes to a load of sodium that for most people is several times over the upper limit for safety.

Adding flavour?

Newborn babies have never tasted salt. It was only when manufacturers of prepared baby foods actually did taste tests with babies, rather than their mothers, that they realised infants favoured foods with no added salt. Once a person's tastebuds become accustomed to a certain level of salt they retain that memory and do not like foods with more or less salt than usual.

It's often said that salt 'brings out the flavour'. Others believe that salt simply adds a salty taste. Once your tastebuds adjust to less salt, you will find heavily salted foods unpleasant and you will also appreciate fresh natural flavours. Gradually cutting back on salt allows your tastebuds to adjust, and after about three months foods you may once have consumed without thought will taste too salty.

You can't always taste salt. Potato crisps taste salty; cornflakes do not, even though they contain more salt.

Iodised salt

Iodine is vital for the functioning of the thyroid gland. Too little or too much of this element can cause the gland to change its activity. During pregnancy and infancy, iodine is especially important for the functioning of the baby's brain. One of Australia's greatest medical researchers, Professor Basil Hetzel, pushed for the introduction of iodised salt in many countries where the lack of iodine in the diet caused severe health problems, greatly reducing the incidence of iodine deficiency throughout the world.

Until a few years ago, most Australians got enough iodine from

167

TIPS FOR USING LESS SALT

- Make full use of herbs and spices (fresh and dried) in your cooking.
- Follow the Greek custom of squeezing lemon juice onto foods. With Asian-style dishes, use lime juice.
- Make sauces using the juices from meat or chicken, adding wine or various types of mustard or vinegar.
- In cool weather, make soups, using lots of fresh vegetables and herbs.
- Choose unsalted products, such as the new range of lentils, chick peas and other canned legumes. Unsalted canned tomatoes, unsalted tomato paste and many other foods without added salt are also available.
- Look for low salt/low sodium products – by law, they must have no more than 120 mg sodium/ 100 g. Products labelled as salt-reduced must have 25 per cent less salt than the standard product, although this still may mean the food is high in salt. Salt-reduced soy sauce, for example, remains extremely high in salt.
- For a snack, choose fruit or unsalted nuts. Enhance the flavour of nuts by toasting them in a dry frying pan over a gentle heat for a few minutes. Cool and store in an airtight container.
- Choose natural muesli or rolled oats or an unsalted breakfast cereal.
- Don't add salt to foods.

dairy products. Some came from the grass the cows ate and some came as a beneficial contaminant from the iodine-containing disinfectants used in dairies. When the makeup of dairy cleansers changed, levels of iodine in milk fell. Mild iodine deficiency has since been found in all areas except Western Australia and Queensland.

Reluctant to recommend that Australians start using iodised salt because it was likely to lead to health problems due to excess sodium, food authorities decided to mandate that all salt used in bread should be iodised. Initial testing in Tasmania found that the practice provided enough iodine to meet the needs of everyone except pregnant women, and the increase in iodine occurred Australia-wide without any increase in the overall salt content of the diet. Most pregnant women are advised to also take an iodine supplement.

Sea salt

Most people think that sea salt is healthier than regular sodium chloride. In fact, analysis shows the average sea salt product is about 84 per cent sodium chloride with moisture making up another 14 per cent or so. The remaining 2 per cent (or less) supposedly consists of about 80 different minerals, but the quantity of any one of them is insignificant. Fortunately, this level of insignificance also applies to the potentially toxic components such as arsenic and strontium found in sea salt.

The larger flakes of sea salt hit the tastebuds and register greater pleasure for most people used to eating added salt. If their more noticeable effect means less sea salt is consumed, that is a possible advantage, but don't kid yourself the product is healthier. When sea salt is dissolved in cooking liquids, the distinctive effect from the large flakes is lost and its use offers no benefits.

Sauces

– add a tasty touch

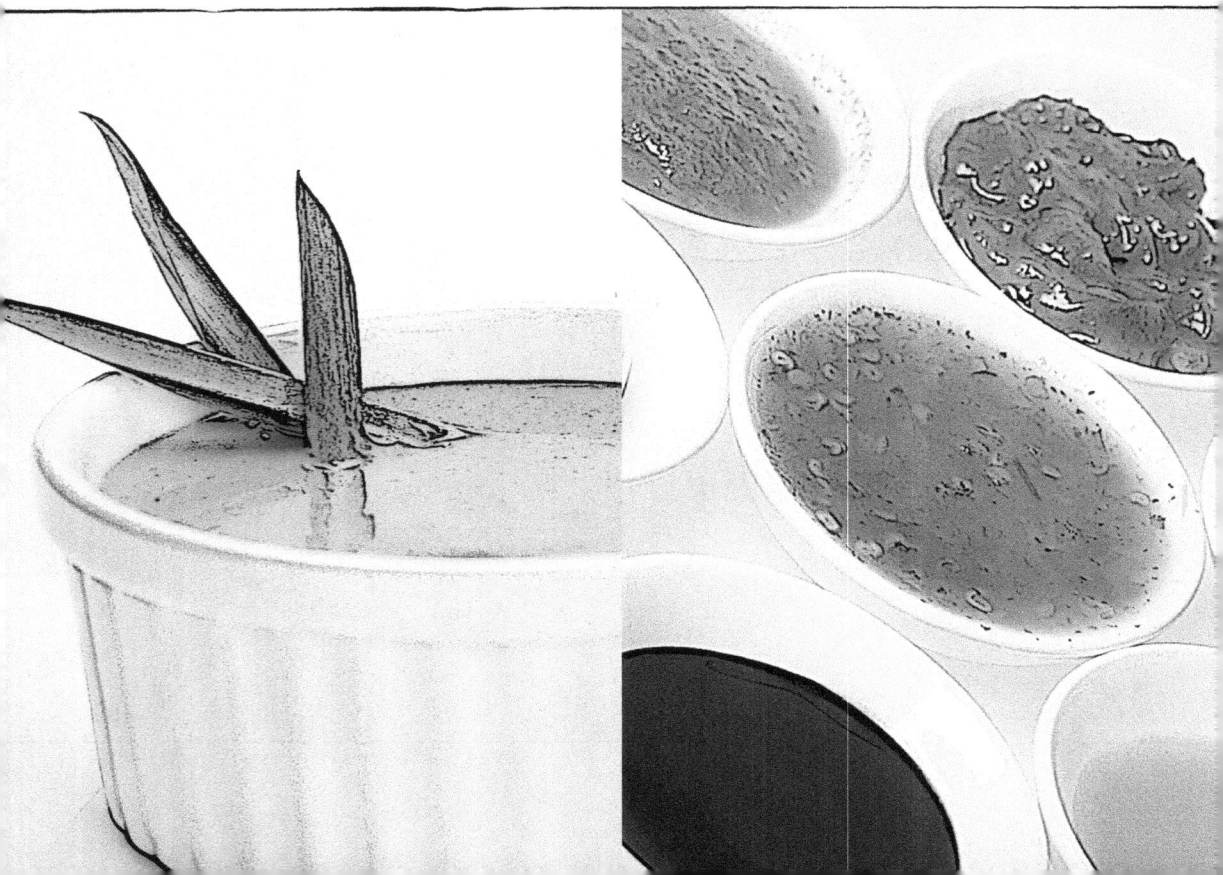

SAUCES ARE UBIQUITOUS IN CUISINES around the world. They vary greatly, but all add flavour and moisture to foods. The first written record of sauces comes from Roman times, when they consisted of the various juices from meats, or wine, flavoured with herbs and thickened with oil and bread beaten into them. These sauces were more a condiment than something to pour over foods. By the 1500s, many cooks used flour instead of bread as the thickener, and herbs and spices were used with restraint and discrimination so that the sauce did not overpower the dish with which it was being served. These days, a whole aisle of the supermarket may be filled with an array of sauces. Some are healthy products, others contain lots of sugar or salt, or both. (This fact may not show up in dietary surveys, because researchers generally fail to include sauces other than tomato sauce.)

Australians were once encouraged to eat cauliflower and other overcooked vegetables by smothering them in a white sauce, made from thickened salted milk with butter and sometimes cheese added. Many people disliked both the vegetables and the sauce! Brown sauces (gravy) werer also thickened with flour.

A range of sauces

Béarnaise is originally from the province of Béarn in France and was first served in 1836 at the opening of a restaurant called Le Pavillon Henri IV. It is made from egg yolks beaten with vinegar, flavoured with peppercorns, bay leaf, tarragon and thyme and thickened with clarified butter. Two tablespoons of a standard home-made recipe has 18 g of fat and 715 kJ.

Béchamel is a white sauce made from butter, flour and milk flavoured with herbs and onion. It is named after Louis de Béchameil, one of Louis XIV's courtiers. Two tablespoons of a standard home-made recipe has approximately 10 g of fat and 465 kJ.

Caramel sauce is a dessert sauce made by caramelising sugar and adding cream or butter. Some varieties are made from sweetened condensed milk. A quarter of a cup of rich caramel sauce has 35 g of fat and 1850 kJ. Ready-made products vary in their fat content and ingredients.

Chilli sauce is a thick hot sauce made from chillies, salt, garlic and

171

vinegar, thickened with some kind of starch. Some sweet chilli sauce has sugar as its main ingredient and may include a range of food additives, including colouring and preservatives. The nutritional content varies, so check the ingredient label.

Fish sauces vary according to their Asian cuisine of origin. Most are made from prawns (including their shells) or small dried or fermented fish. The nutritional value varies with some contributing calcium or iron, but all are high in salt with 1 teaspoon having about 500 mg sodium. Fish sauces usually have very few kilojoules.

Gravy is traditionally made by taking the fat left in the pan used for roasting meat or poultry, adding flour and then either water, stock or wine. Packets of gravy mix consist of modified starches derived from wheat, corn or soy flours, salt, colouring, emulsifiers (to create a smooth texture), hydrolysed protein (usually made from meat or yeast) or MSG (additive 621) or other flavour enhancers, powdered onion or other vegetables, powdered herbs, corn syrup or other sweetener, acids and beef or other fats. Gravy has little positive nutritional value, but values vary according to the recipe. When checking the nutritional value of commercial gravies or gravy powders, note the size of the serving. It may be unrealistically small.

Hoi sin sauce was traditionally made from kumara, but is now made from soy beans, wheat or rice, sugar, vinegar, salt, garlic, chilli and colouring. One tablespoon has about 7 g sugar, some iron, about 320 mg sodium and 200 kJ.

Hollandaise is a rich sauce similar to Béarnaise and originally from Holland. It is made from egg yolks beaten with lemon juice and thickened with butter. Two tablespoons of a standard home-made recipe has 25 g of fat and 950 kJ. Ready-made products or powders generally have less fat and a range of additives.

Mint sauce is traditionally served with roast lamb. It is easily made by pounding a handful of mint in a mortar and pestle with a teaspoon of caster sugar. Add white or wine vinegar and stir and it is ready. It have no fat and makes little contribution apart from flavour. Bought varieties tend to be high in salt.

Mornay sauce is basically béchamel with added cheese. It is the basis of macaroni cheese, popular before Australians started to be more

172

adventurous with pasta. A quarter cup of a standard home-made recipe has approximately 16g of fat and 815 kJ. Commercial mornay sauces sold as dried powders to be reconstituted have less fat and more additives.

Oyster sauce is a dark-coloured sauce made from salted fermented oysters and soy sauce and is widely used in Chinese and other Asian dishes. It does not taste like fish and can be used with beef or chicken. Each tablespoon has about 60 kJ and 460 mg sodium and contributes small amounts of iron.

Peanut sauce, also called *satay sauce*, is often used in Indonesian and Malaysian dishes and is made from ground peanuts, onion, garlic, chilli, shrimp paste, coconut milk and tamarind. A Westernised corruption is often made from peanut butter, onion, tomato and soy sauce. Two tablespoons of home-made peanut sauce has approximately 24 g of fat and 1100 kJ.

Plum sauce is popular with ham, pork or poultry. It is made of plums with onions, sugar, vinegar, cinnamon and pepper, although ready-made versions may also have other additives. Two tablespoons of a home-made recipe has about 135 kJ. Ready-made versions have at least twice as many kilojoules because of their high sugar content.

Soy sauce is made from fermented soy beans, wheat and salt with the recipe differing in various Asian countries. In Japan, soy sauce is also known as shoyu and is made from flakes of soy bean mixed with roasted wheat and a particular strain of yeast and salt. It is left to ferment for a year before being filtered, pasteurised and bottled. Tamari is a soy sauce made from soy beans, usually without wheat, making it suitable for gluten-free diets. Check the label as some brands may contain some wheat. Soy sauce is naturally high in amines and those who have adverse reactions to monosodium glutamate (MSG or additive 621) will often also have adverse reactions to soy sauce, even though it has no added MSG. The major problem with soy sauce is its high salt content. One tablespoon of soy sauce has 1380 mg sodium – more than enough for a whole day. Salt-reduced soy sauce has about half as much sodium, but this is still a high level. Kilojoules are negligible.

Tabasco sauce is a famous hot sauce which uses two varieties of hot peppers (or chillies) originally grown in Tabasco in Mexico. The peppers

173

are ground to a pulp, packed into oak barrels with salt and left for three years. The mixture is then strained and mixed with vinegar and bottled as a thin, very hot sauce. It is used in such small quantities that any nutritional contribution is insignificant.

Tomato sauce is a popular sauce, especially with children. There are two main types of tomato sauce. One (often called passata) is made from fresh or canned tomatoes, onions, herbs and wine (or water) and is used with pasta or as a base for casseroles or other dishes. This is a nutritious product with vitamin C, folate, beta carotene and lycopene from the tomatoes and an average energy content of about 600 kJ/cup. The salt content varies from low to moderate levels. Check the label of different brands. When most people talk of tomato sauce, however, they mean the ubiquitous bottled tomato sauce (known as ketchup in North America) which is made from sugar, tomatoes, vinegar and herbs and spices. One tablespoon contains about a teaspoon of sugar, and has about 90 kJ and 195 mg sodium. Unsalted versions are also available. Used in moderation, tomato sauce is not a problem product, although it can be criticised when some people add it to almost every meal.

Velouté is similar to béchamel but the milk is replaced by fish or chicken stock. Two tablespoons of a standard home-made recipe has approximately 9 g of fat and 410 kJ.

Worcestershire sauce is a sweet-sour dark brown sauce that was first sold commercially in the 1830s in England. It contains a variety of ingredients and was originally made from several varieties of vinegar (including malt vinegar from barley and spirit vinegar), molasses, sugar, salt, anchovies, tamarind extract, onions, garlic, cloves, mace, black and cayenne peppers and lemons. Some varieties also contain soy sauce. The sauce is left to ferment for six months before being pasteurised and bottled. The final product contains some residue, so shake it up before use. It has an extremely long shelf life. Variations of Worcestershire sauce are made in several European countries, North America, Mexico, China and Japan. Some varieties are made without anchovies and are suitable for vegetarians. A gluten-free version is also available. Worcestershire sauce is an ingredient in Welsh rarebit, the drink known as Bloody Mary and in Oysters Kilpatrick. One tablespoon has 250 mg sodium and 75 kJ.

Seeds
– the source of life

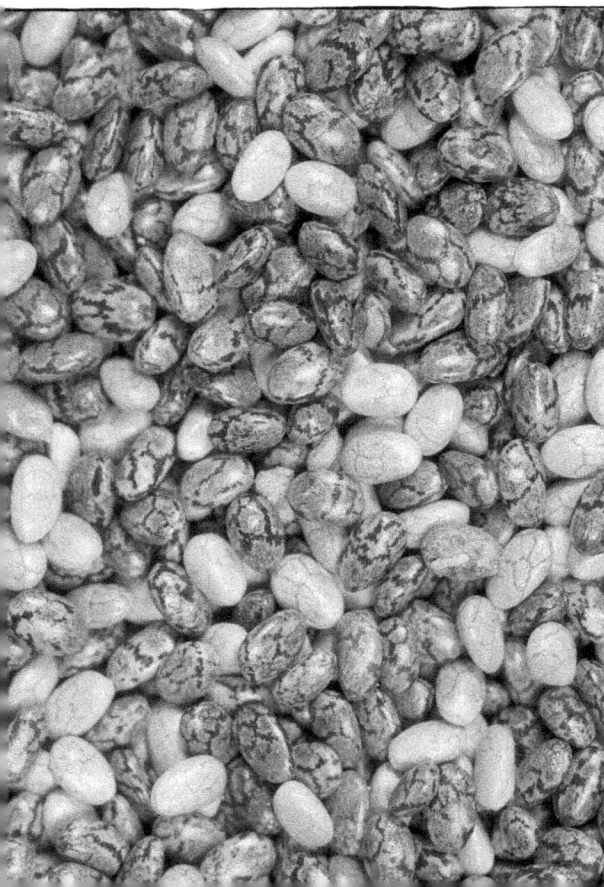

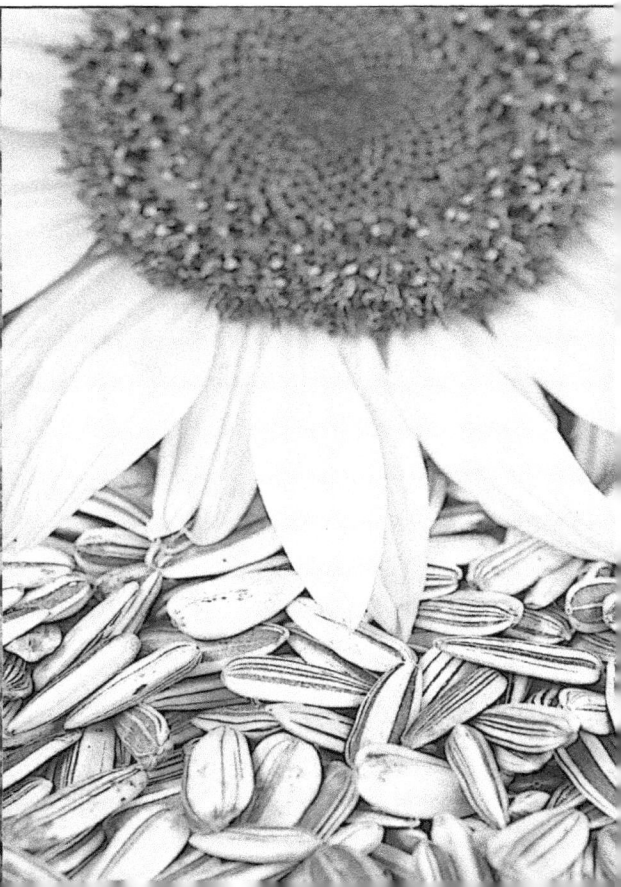

SEEDS ARE UNSUNG HEROES and most people's diets would benefit from their inclusion. They may be small in size, but they pack a powerful nutritional punch. Use them as a snack or add them to muesli and breads, or toast them as a topping for vegetable dishes. The seeds discussed here have no downside and are highly nutritious, either eaten on their own or ground to make pastes such as tahini. However, not all seeds are safe to eat. Apple pips and the seeds within the kernels of apricots, plums and peaches contain some toxic substances, including cyanide.

CHIA

Native to Mexico and Guatemala, chia seeds have long been used in these countries, having been popular with the Aztecs. Australia now rates as the world's greatest producer of chia. The seeds are produced by an annual bush that grows to about 1 metre in height, making harvesting easy. Their current popularity arises because they are a rich source of alpha linolenic acid, an omega 3 fatty acid classified as an essential fat. The seeds can be eaten raw, soaked and made into a porridge or sweet pudding, or ground and added to breads and other baked goods. There is no evidence, however, to support claims the seeds are a super food and studies show no benefits for weight reduction or any ability to reduce inflammation, blood pressure or cholesterol levels. Enjoy them in the knowledge that they are a good source of protein, essential fat and dietary fibre and also contribute some calcium.

LINSEEDS (FLAXSEEDS)

These small brown seeds can be seen in many breads, in muesli and in a mixture known as LSA (linseeds, sunflower seeds and almonds) which is sold in the breakfast cereal aisle. Linseeds are the richest known source of the omega 3 fatty acid, alpha linolenic acid (also found in chia). The rapidly oxidising property of linseed oil gives the oil its familiar use for rubbing into cricket bats and as an ingredient in paints. Unless linseed oil is kept cold from the moment of pressing, it is unlikely to escape randicity.

Because the hard brown seed coat protects the delicate fats within from oxidation, it is better to eat the seeds rather than trying to use the

176

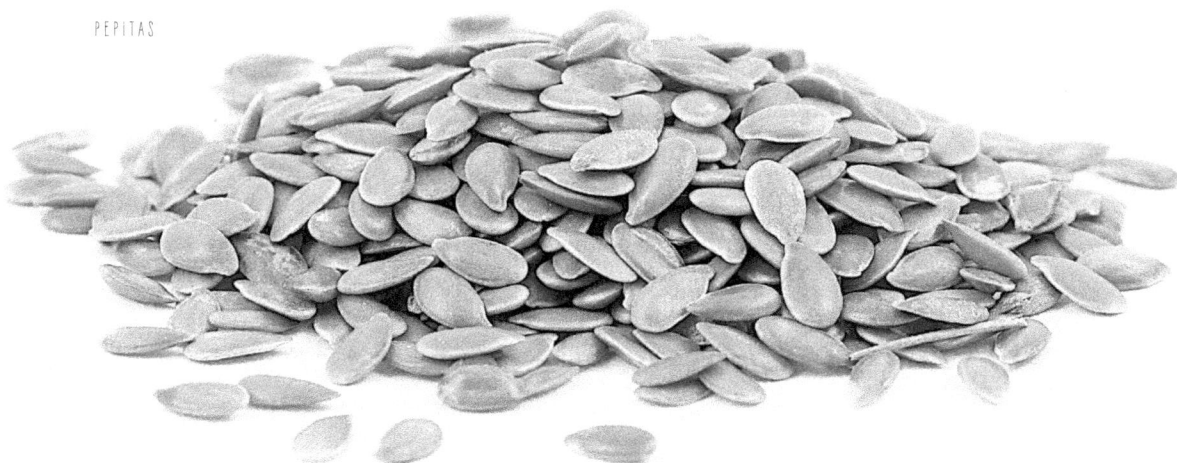

oil. Some of the seeds will be digested, some stick to the wall of the bowel and some are passed intact. This is not a problem and the seeds on the wall of the bowel are gradually digested by 'good' bacteria. (People who require a colonoscopy must avoid linseeds for 10–12 days beforehand, as the seeds can damage the delicate instrument used for the examination.) As well as providing a valuable fatty acid, linseeds are a good source of protein, dietary fibre, calcium, iron, zinc, selenium, potassium, magnesium and vitamin E. They are also rich in lutein and zeaxanthin, two carotenoids that promote eye health.

PEPITAS

These green pumpkin seed kernels are a top source of vitamin E and also provide iron, zinc, magnesium, potassium, protein, dietary fibre and some of the B complex vitamins. Their fat is mostly the healthy unsaturated kind, so enjoy them as a snack, in muesli or on top of steamed cauliflower.

POPPY

These tiny black or white seeds come from the opium poppy, but they have no narcotic properties since the fluid which forms the opium is only present in the bud before the seeds form. The poppy is native to Greece, and has spread far and wide around the world. The seeds have been used since prehistoric times. White poppy seeds are used in Indian cooking.

177

Black seeds are popular in breads, cakes and in Jewish cuisine. Even in the modest quantities likely to be consumed, poppy seeds supply calcium, some iron and dietary fibre. Like all seeds, their fat is unsaturated.

SAFFLOWER

These crunchy seeds come from an annual flowering plant that is native to parts of Asia and Africa. Safflower is grown commercially in Australia, mainly for the polyunsaturated oil in its seeds. Eating the safflower seeds would make more sense, since they provide dietary fibre, protein and a selection of minerals and vitamins, including vitamin E.

SESAME

Black and white varieties of sesame seeds are among the world's oldest cultivated crops, probably originating in Morocco or India. Ali Baba and the forty thieves obviously attributed mystical powers to sesame seeds – hence 'open sesame'. Egyptian tomb paintings from at least 2000 BC depict bakers adding the seeds to bread dough, and they have been part of the cuisines of China, Korea and Japan (where they are known as goma) for at least 5000 years. They are valued for the intense flavour of their oil, which keeps well because of its high content of natural antioxidants. Folklore also claims that they increase virility.

Sesame seeds can be added to breads, biscuits and cakes, or toasted and used with vegetable dishes, in muesli or as a coating for various foods in place of (or with) breadcrumbs. They can also be ground into tahini paste. Sesame seeds are rich in vitamin E, and supply dietary fibre, protein, zinc and iron, but they provide less calcium than is popularly believed because the seed husk contains oxalates that bind calcium and makes it unavailable for absorption.

SUNFLOWER

Native to North America, the sunflower was taken to Europe as a decorative plant. By the eighteenth century, sunflowers were being grown in France and parts of Germany for their seeds and their oil. Sunflowers are now widely cultivated and their oil is used in margarines or as a frying oil. The seeds themselves are high in protein and dietary fibre and a good source of minerals, including iron. Their fat is largely polyunsaturated.

Snacks
– sweet and savoury

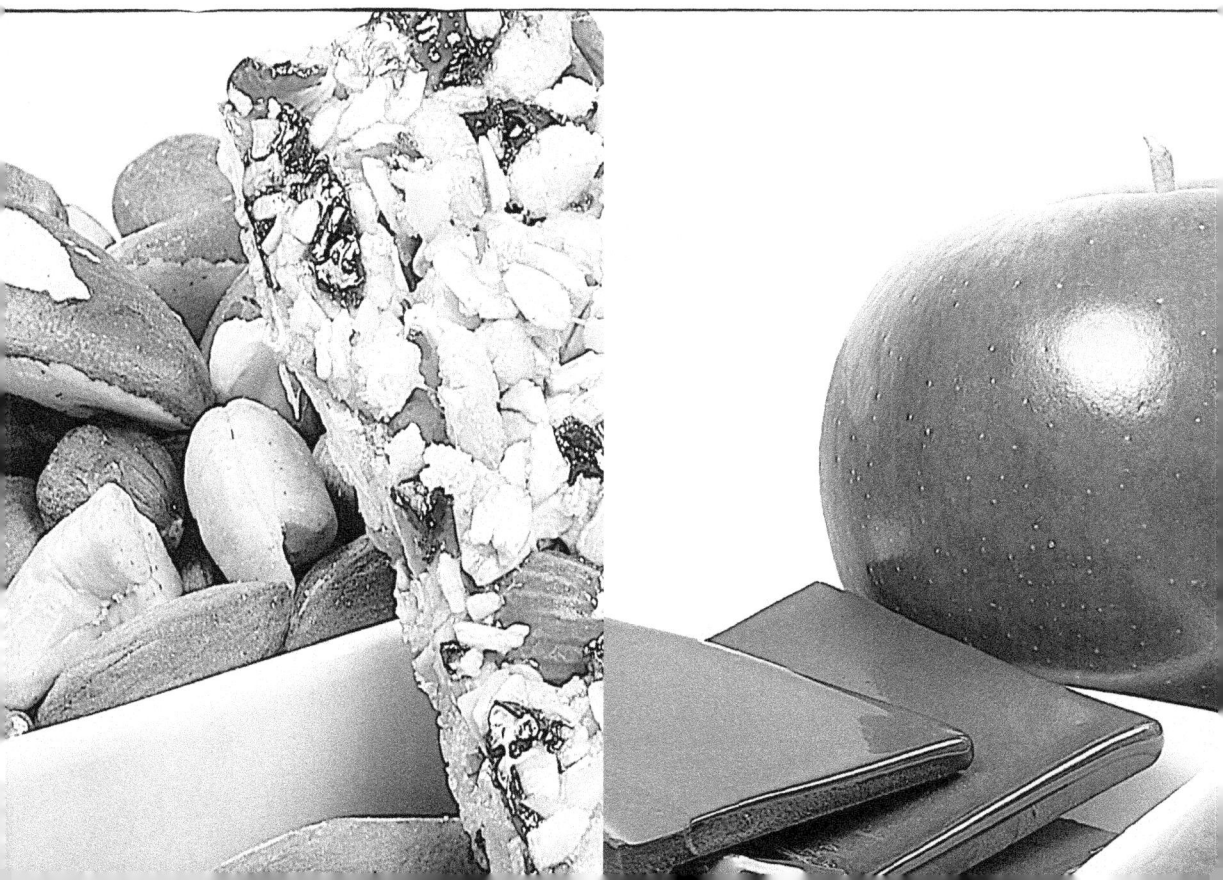

THE AVERAGE SUPERMARKET now carries about 1800 different snack foods. When we pay for fuel for our cars we are confronted by dozens of snack foods. At train stations, and in many office buildings and hospitals, vending machines are strategically placed to tempt us. Most of their offerings are largely fat with sugar or fat with salt. Few healthy options are available.

When a group of food marketers once asked me what I would consider to be a healthy snack and I replied 'fruit', I was told that fruit wasn't a snack. I asked why and was told that it didn't qualify because it didn't come in a packet! Packeted snack foods now make up a large part of the diet for many people. A few make a worthwhile contribution to the diet, but most can be classified as junk foods. Nutritionists generally define junk foods as those that contribute kilojoules, but have few (if any) essential nutrients. Other definitions include foods that contain some nutritious ingredients but also have a large quantity of added fat, salt or sugar, like chicken nuggets and many fast foods.

In the average Australian adult's diet, 36 per cent of the kilojoules come from food and drinks that are not included in the five food groups (see Healthy eating, page 10). For children, the percentage rises to over 40 per cent. Few would dispute that some of our day's energy can come from foods that are not healthy enough to be part of the food groups, but the current proportion is absurdly high in a population where the majority (62 per cent) of adults and a quarter of children are too fat. Snacks need some attention.

Who needs snacks?

Most people's nutritional needs will be met by three meals a day. Snacks may be important for the small children who find it hard to sit at the table long enough to eat enough to last them until the following meal. But it is also easy for small children to get into the habit of rejecting foods offered at mealtimes, then filling up on snacks between meals so that they are not hungry enough for the next meal. This 'vicious circle' is an unhealthy way of eating and is best avoided. Parents can take comfort in the fact that no healthy child ever starved when food was available, even if it is only available at mealtimes.

Active growing children and adolescents and anyone engaging in vigorous activity lasting more than an hour or two may need to eat more than three times a day, but growth and activity require nutrients, not just kilojoules, so a snack between meals needs to be healthy. Few people, whatever their level of activity, need to eat more than once between meals.

Food also plays a social role for most of us and may involve eating between meals. Again, if this involves eating more than once between meals, we need to make changes.

How often?

The idea that frequent snacking will stimulate metabolism and help with weight loss has recently been debunked. Earlier studies claiming that small and often was a better way to eat always involved snacks being provided along with smaller meals. In real life, when people are left to choose their own meals and snacks, few reduce the size of their meals enough to accommodate the kilojoules from their snacks. For those who like eating small and often, the easiest way to do this healthily is to save half (or part) or a meal to eat midway between that meal and the next, or a couple of hours later in the case of the evening meal.

Eating often is a major problem for dental health. Normally, over the couple of hours after we have eaten, minerals in saliva act to neutralise compounds that contribute to decay. Eating frequently interrupts this vital function. Dentists believe that the increase in decay is due to more frequent snacking. Any food containing carbohydrate has the potential to be especially attractive to bacteria in the mouth that cause decay. Potato crisps or crackers can be as much of a problem for teeth as sweet biscuits. Although fruit contains natural sugars, it is less of a problem because it stimulates extra production of protective saliva. Sipping acidic drinks, including diet soft drinks, also contributes to the erosion of the enamel on teeth.

Ideally, those who snack should ensure they keep to one snack between meals.

181

Which snack?

In school canteens and some government institutions, foods are now rated as green (suitable for every day), yellow (take care as there may be high levels of salt, sugar or saturated fat accompanying the valuable nutrients present) or red (no real nutritional value, or high in sugar, fat or salt). A recent labelling review (2011) recommends a similar 'traffic light labelling system' should be applied to foods sold in supermarkets. The system has several advantages. It makes for easier shopping without having to study and interpret food labels and also gives some idea of how often foods should be consumed. No food needs to be banned, but some should only be consumed occasionally.

Green-light snacks

Foods in this category have a good nutritional profile, but moderation is the key with snacks, as with foods eaten at any time.

FRUIT

A piece of fresh fruit is a healthy food whenever it is consumed, but eating fruit more than once between meals can diminish the protection that saliva usually provides. It is better to eat two pieces of fruit at the one time than to have two separate fruit snacks between adjacent meals. If more food is needed during an active sport session, rinse your mouth with plain water after eating.

Dried fruit can stick between the teeth, although often an older child or adult will notice this and take steps to remove the bits. Dried fruits are a much healthier choice than lollies, but nibbling on dried fruit over several hours can increase the risk of dental decay.

VEGETABLES

A radio presenter once asked me if I thought it was a good idea for a parent to take a small container of carrots and celery for the children to nibble on their car journey on the way home from school. I don't doubt the value of vegetables, but I think it would be even better for the children to wait until they got home. For a short journey, children don't need food, and pairing snacking with another activity, such as getting into the car, encourages excess consumption in both children and adults. Why not wait until you get home to enjoy some carrot sticks or celery or snow peas or cherry tomatoes?

YOGHURT

An excellent food, with its calcium, protein, riboflavin, vitamin B12 and (depending on the brand) potentially useful 'good' bacteria, yoghurt makes an excellent snack. In most households, the most economical and most environmentally friendly way to enjoy yoghurt is to buy a large container and spoon smaller quantities into re-usable containers. These can be enjoyed at home or packed into the lunchbox next to a bottle of frozen water. Special 'baby' or children's yoghurts are unnecessary and most cost more and are too high in sugar to rate highly. Natural and Greek yoghurt (which is drained so it is thicker and creamier) are ideal. Add fresh fruit if you prefer a sweeter product. If buying flavoured yoghurt, check the ingredient list and the nutrition information panel as some brands, especially reduced-fat varieties, have large amounts of added sugar.

SMOOTHIES

Home-made smoothies are ideal for children and adolescents as they combine milk and yoghurt (both good sources of calcium and other nutrients) with fresh or frozen fruit. To make a smoothie, combine a cup of reduced-fat milk, a spoonful of yoghurt, fruit (banana, frozen berries, mango or melon) and blend until thick and frothy. Adding ice cubes is good in summer and makes the smoothie extra frothy. When bananas are cheap, or if they are likely to be left because the skin is starting to show flecks of colour, peel them and freeze ready for making a smoothie later on.

Some commercially available smoothies are high in sugar and that fact, combined with their large size, means that even those listed as 'low fat' may have 2000 kJ.

NUTS

As discussed on pages 144–152, nuts are a healthy choice. In general, the amount that fits easily into the palm of your hand is about the right amount for a snack. Choose unsalted nuts for preference, but if only salted nuts are available, leave the salt that falls to the bottom of the packet.

TRAIL MIX

A combination of nuts, seeds (pepitas, sunflower) and dried fruits is an excellent snack for those who need plenty of kilojoules in a compact form. The name gives the clue for hikers, but cross-country skiers, cyclists, kayakers and other endurance enthusiasts need snack foods too, and trail mix is ideal. Either mix your own or check the ingredient list on ready-mixed products.

'BREAKFAST' CEREALS

Wholewheat breakfast biscuits are a popular choice for children (or active adults) to have as a between-meal snack. Other wholegrain cereals are also good choices.

ENGLISH MUFFINS

Made from a dough similar to bread, English muffins have a similar nutritional profile to bread. Choose wholemeal muffins for the best fibre level.

CRUMPETS

Popular in England, crumpets are made from a yeasted batter cooked on a hot plate to give a smooth surface on one side and a holey appearance on the other. When toasted, the holey side is spread with butter and honey or yeast extract, but because the melted butter falls through easily, the total amount used may be less than it appears – and the crumpet itself has virtually no fat. Wholemeal crumpets provide some dietary fibre.

CHEESE

Some cheese sticks are so high in salt that they can't be considered a green light food and so must be moved to the yellow light category. Regular cheese is fine and some stringy cheese sticks have more calcium and less than half the high salt content of regular cheese sticks. They also have less fat and no additives. Cheese cut into animal shapes is also designed to appeal to children and has more fat than cheese strings but less salt. Cheese is a good source of calcium and if children are happy with a single stringy stick or one animal shape, they pass as a suitable snack food.

CRACKERS

Some crackers have low levels of fat, are made with whole grains (usually wheat or rye) and may include small quantities of sesame or other seeds. The only potential negative for these products is their salt content, but even here reduced-salt varieties are available. These crackers or crispbread are at the green end of the snack spectrum. Those who mistakenly think of bread as a fattening food often turn to crackers, but spreads or other toppings used on their large surface area wipe out any potential savings in kilojoules.

Rice crackers have little positive nutritional value, but they are low in fat and their salt content is usually lower than other crackers.

Flaky crackers made with white flour tend to have little to offer and have over 20 per cent fat with about half that either saturated or trans fat. Their salt content is also high and these products move towards the red end of the snack spectrum.

Water crackers and similar plain crackers have about half the fat of flaky crackers, but make little positive or negative contribution. For children, their fine starch can stick in the teeth and promote decay.

HOME-POPPED CORN

If you like popcorn, you may be following an old tradition, since archaeologists in New Mexico have unearthed popped corn dating back to 3500 BC. Not all varieties of corn are suitable for popping. The popping process requires kernels with about 12 per cent moisture. Corn contains protein and starch and when the dried kernels are heated, the moisture starts to gelatinise the starch. As the temperature increases inside the grain, the water expands and exerts pressure on the protein, bursting the kernel and allowing the centre section (the endosperm) to expand. At the same time, the gelatinised starch dries out, leaving a dry, crisp, popped piece of corn.

Home-popped corn, made with a hot air popper or popped in a large saucepan on the stove with a small amount of oil, is a healthy alternative to high-fat savoury snacks. It provides dietary fibre and some beta

185

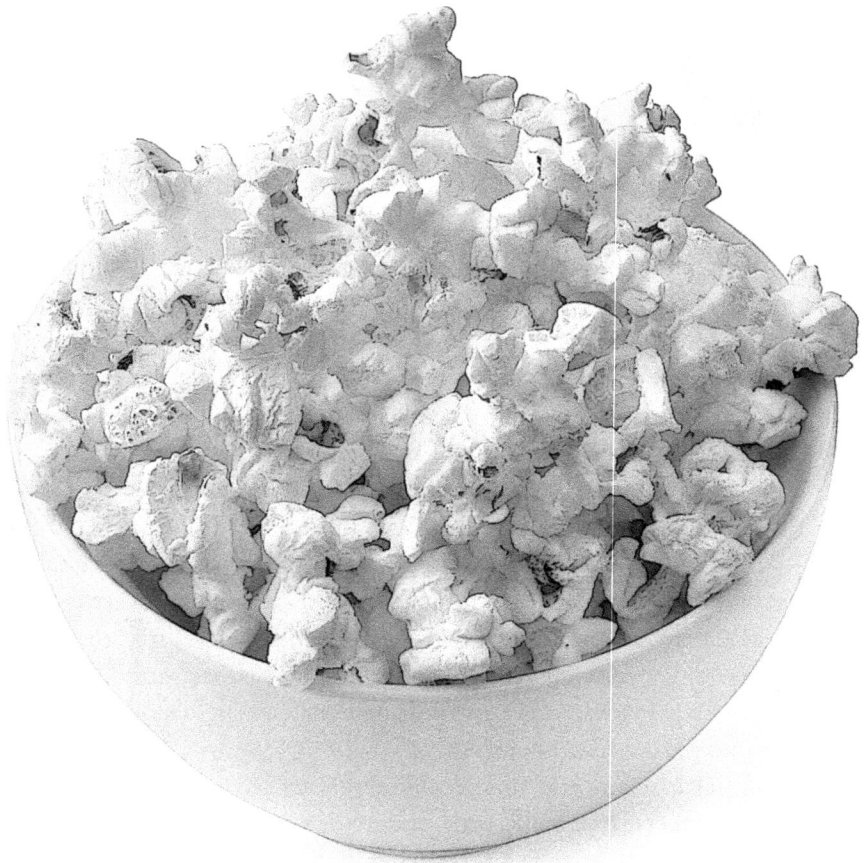

carotene, has very little fat and is low in kilojoules, as long as you don't add lots of butter. Instead of adding salt, sprinkle the popped corn with dried parsley or a mixture of freshly ground pepper and a touch of chilli powder. A 100 g packet of corn kernels will make about 12 cups of popcorn. Commercial popcorn and corn ready to pop in the microwave are a different story and fit into the red light snacks.

Yellow-light snacks

Foods in this category contain some nutrients, but may have higher levels of fat, salt or sugar.

CHEESE STICKS

Made from processed cheese, the traditional cheese stick contains a range of additives, including emulsifiers, preservatives and food acids.

None of these is harmful, but all can be avoided by eating regular cheese or stringy cheese sticks, both of which have a lower salt content than regular cheese sticks. However, cheese sticks do provide calcium and protein and so they fit into the yellow light category

PIKELETS

Made from a batter containing flour, a raising agent, milk, eggs and a small amount of sugar, pikelets are cooked in a hot pan and are sometimes thought of as an Australian version of a griddle cake. From a nutritional perspective, they have no special virtues or vices and are usually small enough to provide a modest kilojoule count.

SCONES

Known as biscuits in the United States, scones are made from a soft dough of self-raising flour, milk and a small amount of butter. They are best eaten soon after baking. A pot of tea served with scones, jam and cream is known as a Devonshire tea. Like pikelets, scones are nutritionally fairly neutral and an average scone has about 460 kJ.

Red-light snacks – sweet and savoury

Foods listed here have little positive nutritional value. All these foods should be kept to a minor place in the diet. Some are probably best avoided because their saltiness or sweetness can teach the tastebuds bad habits. When these foods are eaten daily or dominate the diet at any time, other healthy foods are either decreased or the total amount of food increases. With the majority of adults and a quarter of children now overweight or obese, the average person needs to cut consumption of these foods. For children, try using the term 'sometimes' foods; with pre-schoolers, you will need to define 'sometimes', since children that age tend to think 'sometimes' is right now. 'Sometimes' may be once a week.

SWEET SNACKS

Some sweet snack foods have some goodness and if it wasn't for their high sugar content and stickiness could earn a yellow light (meaning 'enjoy occasionally').

MUESLI BARS

The main ingredient in muesli is oats, a wholegrain cereal that deserves a tick. Most muesli bars, however, contain only small quantities of oats and their ingredients are dominated by various types of sugar. Using two or more types of sugar means that each form of sugar can move down the ingredient list, even though the total sugar content may be high enough to make it the major ingredient. For this reason, beware of products that include more than one type of sugar. Most muesli bars also contain fat, which may be saturated fat. Nuts and seeds are also healthy ingredients, but most bars contain minimal quantities, especially the cheaper ones. Check the ingredient list on any muesli bar. There may be exceptions, but in general, the more ingredients, the lower the nutritional value. Skip any that contain humectants, emulsifiers, acids, preservatives and added flavours, which may be unidentified but described as 'natural'. It is not so much the additives that are a problem but that their presence usually indicates the bar contains minimum quantities of 'real' ingredients and more fillers, sugars and fats. Remember too that you tend to get what you pay for so the cheaper bars are likely to have less of the whole grains, fruit, nuts and seeds and more junk. Don't forget to check the size as well. A large muesli bar may contain a whole meal's worth of kilojoules, but with only a small fraction of the nutrients required.

Muesli bars have a possible role for those on extended hikes or other endurance pursuits where packing plenty of kilojoules into a small space is important. Just remember to pack your toothbrush or at least have a good rinse with plain water.

BREAKFAST CEREAL BARS

To turn a breakfast cereal into a cereal bar, you need to add plenty of sugar, and usually some fat, although most cereal bars have less fat than muesli bars. Nonetheless, some breakfast bars rate as having the highest content of trans fat (over 30 per cent) of any foods tested. No level of industrially produced trans fat can be considered safe. The sugar in these products dilutes any dietary fibre and most other nutrients that were present in the original cereal. And without the milk that is added to a bowl of cereal, a cereal bar is a poor substitute for breakfast.

Breakfast cereals vary and so do cereal bars that bear their names.

188

Almost without exception, cereal bars have at least 35 per cent sugar, which is up to three times the quantity in some of the cereals themselves. Most cereal bars use different types of sugars, including sucrose (ordinary sugar), glucose as glucose syrup or glucose solids or dextrose, raw sugar, brown sugar, malt extract (or maltose), fructose and honey. The fibre content may be negligible or, in bars made from higher fibre cereal grains, the fibre is usually half the original level. Some products have more sugar and fat than chocolate confectionery. Check the ingredients and the size of the serve, and look at them as confectionery rather than a breakfast option.

FRUIT BARS

Often featuring pictures of strawberries, apricots, apples or pears, fruit bars usually contain very little of the featured fruit. Some bars are labelled as 100 per cent fruit, but a closer inspection reveals that the fruit is usually concentrated pear or apple juice. Pears and apples are nutritious, high fibre fruits, but their concentrated juice is little more than sugar.

The 'fruit' may also have little resemblance to anything that grew on a fruit tree. In one product, the 'strawberry' contained just over 2 per cent strawberry puree with the rest of it listed as apple paste, pear paste, plum paste, invert sugar, sugar, humectant, wheat fibre, gelling agent, malic acid and elderberry flavouring. Other ingredients in the 'fruit' in some products include maltodextrins, fructose (fruit sugar), vegetable gums, vegetable fat (which may contain trans fat) and firming agents.

These products are not substitutes for fruit and are particularly bad for dental health as they are missing most of the dietary fibre of the original fruit. The quality of fruit bars varies between brands, but none is equivalent to eating fresh fruit and they do not count as a serving of fruit in dietary guideline recommendations. Nothing need be forbidden in a healthy diet, but most of these products are simply confectionery masquerading as a healthy food.

SWEET BISCUITS

Sugar, saturated fat, refined flours and starches are the major ingredients in sweet biscuits. A few, such as Anzac biscuits, have some added oats and some have a small quantity of dried fruit, but sweet biscuits fit firmly into the category of 'extras' providing kilojoules but virtually no

189

nutritional goodies. Large American-style cookies can have enough kilojoules for an entire meal, but without the nutrients you need, so unless you also want a big round middle, find some friends to share if you are tempted by one of these giant discs of sugar and fat. Biscuits don't work with unsaturated fat – they go soggy. Commercial bakers use either saturated fat or trans fat. There is currently no legal requirement in Australia for trans fat to be labelled, so it's a case of buyer beware. The ingredient list should give you a clue by including partially hydrogenated oil, but even that is not required so it will probably simply say vegetable oil.

MUFFINS AND CAKES

English muffins have a similar nutrient profile to bread. Cake-like muffins are nutritionally similar to cakes – often very large cakes. Some commercial muffins have half a day's supply of fat and about 35 per cent of an average woman's kilojoules. The belief that bran or blueberry muffins are somehow healthy is a rationalisation. Their content of healthy ingredients is usually dwarfed by their fat, sugar and kilojoules. Look for smaller muffins or share a large one.

DONUTS

High in fat (often in the form of trans fat) and with little positive nutritional contribution, donuts are made from a yeasted sweet dough. They have a high fat content and fit firmly in the red light category. Most donuts have between 1400 and 1800 kJ and about half their fat is saturated or trans fat.

CROISSANTS AND PASTRIES

With the exception of filo, pastry is high in fat. The best-tasting croissants and pastries are made with butter. A smallish croissant is a delicious treat. A larger croissant has about the same kilojoule and fat count as 4 thick slices of buttered toast. Croissants can be accommodated as an occasional treat, but eating one or two for breakfast each morning may leave a lasting legacy.

SAVOURY SNACKS

Often considered 'healthier' than sweet snacks, remember that the highly refined carbohydrate in these foods is ideal food for the bacteria that cause tooth decay.

CORN CHIPS

With slightly less fat and salt than potato crisps and twice as much fibre, corn chips are a better choice. Reduced-salt versions are available in the health food section and could possibly move to the yellow category.

EXTRUDED SNACK FOODS

High in fat (>31 g/100 g), with half of that in the form of saturated fat, these crunchy, puffy, often air-filled savoury snacks are also very high in sodium. Take claims such as 'contains all the goodness of cheese' with a grain of salt (actually several grains), since the cheese content is minuscule and far too low to offer any nutritional benefits. Check the ingredient list for additives – often two or three different flavour enhancers, three or four different food acids, lots of salt and colouring. These are suitable only for an occasional party food and even then, I would try to avoid them mainly to avoid giving children a taste for artificial junk foods. They have no redeeming nutritional qualities and their fine starch is hazardous for teeth.

POPCORN

Air-popped corn or home-popped corn is included in the green light list. Microwave popcorn doesn't fit there as it is high in fat, saturated fat and salt, with a single pack having more fat than a chocolate bar. A bucket of popcorn bought at the movies may contain 13 cups of popcorn with about 30 g of fat and 2260 kJ and a whole day's salt. If you buy it, find plenty of friends for sharing.

POTATO CRISPS

Potatoes are a nutritious food, but their starchy carbohydrate soaks up fat and when they are sliced finely for potato crisps they soak up a *lot* of fat. Although crisps are cooked in oil, about a third of their fat is saturated, indicating that the oil has been hydrogenated or is a more highly saturated product such as palm oil. Some brands of crisps also contain trans fat from partially hydrogenated oil, with some having over 20 per cent trans fat. No level of industrially produced trans fat is considered safe, although some countries accept a level up to 1–2 per cent. Crisps are high in total fat, saturated fat and salt, but they do provide some vitamins C and E.

Beware of 'light' crisps. They may be lighter in salt or simply sliced more finely. Most have similar fat and kilojoule levels to regular crisps.

Soups
and stocks

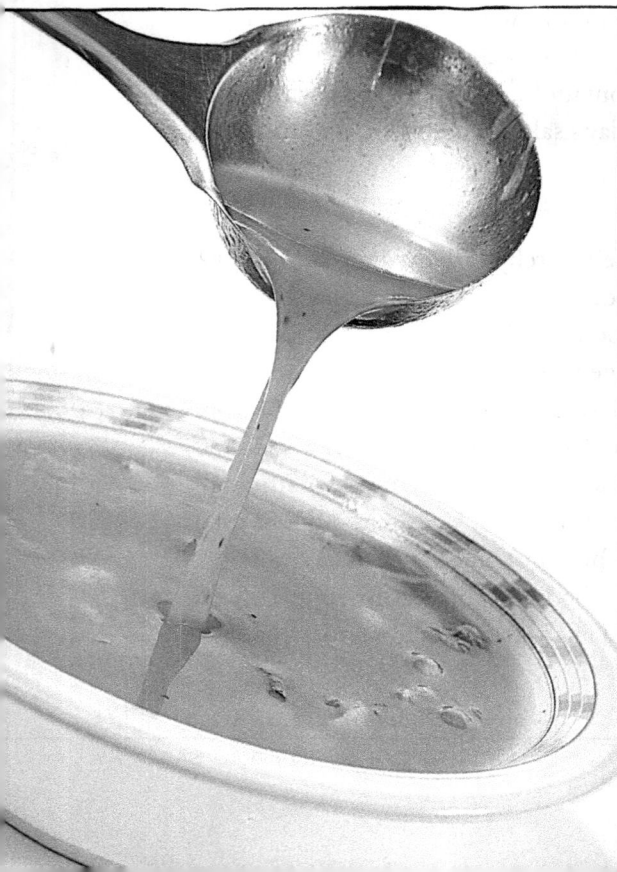

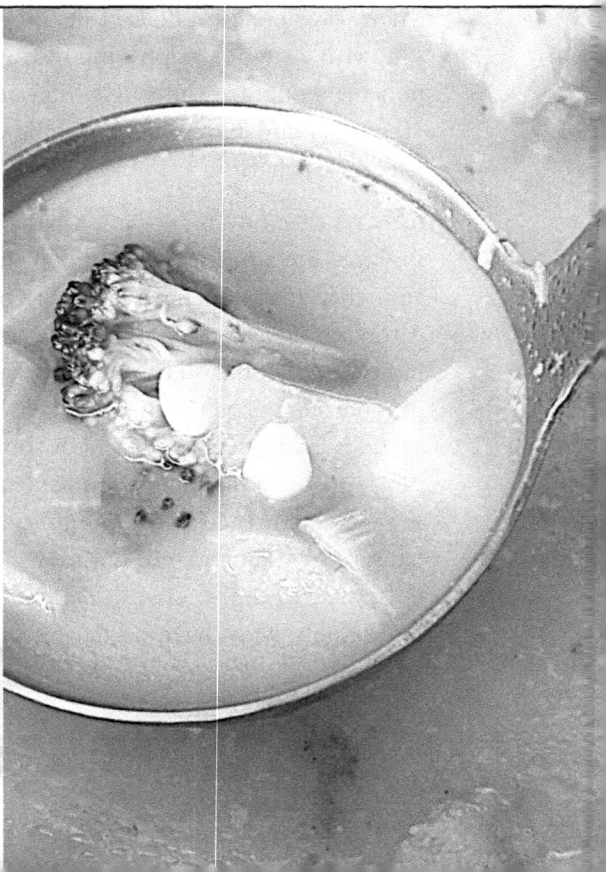

SOUPS CAN BE WONDERFULLY WARMING winter foods or chilled and refreshing in the heat of summer. Soups are also filling, can be frozen, and reheated from their frozen state on the stove top or in a microwave oven. Soups are easy to make and home-made soups are likely to be more nutritious than canned and packet soups available in the supermarket. Before buying a ready-made soup or a powdered product, check the ingredient list – you may be paying for salt, flavour enhancers and a range of other additives with little nutritional worth.

Stocks

A stock is basically a liquid made by extracting the flavour from seafood, meat, chicken or vegetables. A brown stock is made by roasting the bones or vegetables and then boiling the roasted ingredients with water, herbs and fresh vegetables such as onion, carrot and celery. Roasted chicken bones and carcasses make an excellent brown stock. A white stock is made without browning the bones. Stocks made using chicken and veal bones contain collagen and set to a flavoursome jelly when they are refrigerated. Jellied stock is ideal for deglazing a baking dish or frying pan as you stir to dislodge the flavoursome 'bits' to add to sauces and gravies. Any kind of stock is useful in making risotto, soups and sauces.

According to the elite foodie bible, *Larousse Gastronomique*, stock should not be salty since seasoning should wait until a sauce or dish is 'perfected'. Liquid stock, stock cubes and powders are all high in salt. Those labelled as salt-reduced still contain a large amount of salt and are unsuitable for anyone seeking to control high blood pressure.

Make your own

CHICKEN STOCK

Place chicken carcasses or bones, a roughly chopped onion, a stick of celery and half a sliced lemon in an oiled roasting pan and bake in a moderate oven for 30 minutes. Tip the bones into a saucepan, add a handful of fresh herbs (thyme, parsley, rosemary), a dozen black peppercorns, 1.5 L water, bring to the boil, cover and simmer for 1 hour. Strain and refrigerate or freeze.

VEAL STOCK

Ask the butcher to saw a veal shank into several pieces. Into a large saucepan, place the shank, a roughly sliced onion, a stick or two of celery, 4–6 bay leaves, some peppercorns, a few stalks of parsley, some fresh or dried thyme and 1.5 L water. Bring to the boil, cover and simmer for 2 hours. Strain stock into a bowl and refrigerate or freeze. The meat from the veal bones can be removed and used in a soup, if desired.

VEGETABLE STOCK

Heat 1 tablespoon of olive oil in a saucepan, add a chopped onion, 2 cloves garlic, fresh herbs and peppercorns (as for chicken stock) and cook for 3–4 minutes, stirring often. Add 1.5 L water and about 6 cups of roughly chopped unpeeled vegetables (celery, carrot, leek, mushrooms, tomatoes, zucchini). Bring to the boil, cover and simmer for 1 hour. Strain and refrigerate or freeze.

FISH STOCK

Place the bones and head of a fish and/or some prawn shells into a saucepan with a roughly chopped onion, a stalk or two of sliced celery, carrot and herbs, 1 L of water and 1 cup of white wine (optional). Bring to the boil, cover and simmer for no more than 15 minutes. Strain and refrigerate or freeze.

TO CLARIFY STOCK

Clarified stock is a clear stock used to make a consommé or a savoury jelly. To clarify 1.5 L stock, place it into a saucepan, add a chopped carrot and a stick of sliced celery and the beaten whites of two eggs. Stir the stock mixture until it boils, turn the heat very low and simmer for about 45 minutes. Scoop the egg white from the surface and strain the liquid through fine cheesecloth into a bowl. Refrigerate, and use within 2–3 days. Clarified stock can also be frozen.

Stock	Sodium content (mg)
Home-made (unsalted), 1 cup	100
Stock powder, 2 teaspoons	800–1800
Stock cube, 1 small (3.3 g)	350–900
Liquid stock, chicken, 1 cup	1300*
Liquid stock, chicken, salt-reduced, 1 cup	640*
Liquid stock, vegetable, 1 cup	1370*
Liquid stock, vegetable, salt-reduced, 1 cup	1025*
Liquid stock, beef, 1 cup	1270*
Liquid stock, beef, salt-reduced, 1 cup	1000*

* Average value. Some brands may have more or less, so check the label.

Soups

ARE THEY GOOD FOR YOU?

A soup is only as nutritious as what goes into it. I was amused some years ago when a food technologist was discussing the difficulties of making canned soups without added salt. I offered to give him my recipe for pumpkin soup. I start by roasting the pumpkin, a large onion and some garlic, because roasting caramelises some of the natural sugars in the vegetables and provides more flavour. I put the roasted vegetables into a saucepan with some herbs and spices, add home-made stock to the roasting pan to soak off the flavoursome 'bits' and then pour this into my saucepan. After about 10 minutes or so of simmering, I remove the bay leaves I've used, and puree the soup, adding powdered skim milk or reduced-fat milk if I want it to be creamy. I don't add salt. When next I saw him, the food technologist remarked that my recipe didn't work. I quizzed him about the quality of his stock and the herbs and

195

spices he had used. The crunch came when I asked if he had roasted the pumpkin and he told me he couldn't possibly use the large amount of pumpkin in my recipe – so he'd used some pumpkin powder instead. I repeat the story because it shows why canned and packet soups have so much salt and other additives – it's because they use very little of the 'real' ingredient.

If you have a vegetable garden, you are undoubtedly aware of how easy it is to over-produce some vegies. Zucchini, cauliflower, broccoli, potatoes, tomatoes, spinach and many other vegetables that home gardeners grow tend to produce with gay abundance. Using them to make soup and freezing portions for later use makes good sense. It is also a way to get lots of vegies into reluctant vegetable eaters!

The answer to winter weight gain may lie in soup. Many studies have reported that when we consume sugar-sweetened drinks, the body does not register the kilojoules, and we continue to eat as much as we do when we drink water. Soup seems to be different – several studies show that, unlike sweet drinks, soup is filling, decreases hunger and helps people eat less. Researchers suggest that different characteristics of soup may be responsible for its filling qualities, including the amount consumed, the hot temperature or the viscosity of the soup.

A recent study gave volunteers a standard breakfast and at lunchtime presented them (on different days) with different soups made from identical ingredients – a clear broth with vegetables added just before serving, a chunky vegetable soup, a soup with half the vegetables pureed into it and the rest stirred through, and a totally smooth pureed vegetable soup. After the soup, the participants were given a regular meal, but were unaware that how much they ate was being measured. After consuming the soup, the participants all ate less of the food on offer. The form of the soup had no influence and when the energy from the soup and the food eaten was added up, the total number of kilojoules consumed was less than when no soup was provided.

READ THE LABEL

Before buying a soup, read the ingredients, noting that they must be listed in descending order of prominence in the product. Some chicken soups have less than 1 per cent chicken. Other soups have such a range of additives to enhance flavour or keep fat emulsified, and so much salt, that you can easily work out that they have little of the real ingredient on offer.

The extra price of refrigerated fresh soups probably reflects the fact that most have more of real food ingredients. Check their sodium level and choose those with the lowest levels. The sodium content is one test of quality.

SOUP AS A MEAL

Soups that contain plenty of vegetables plus legumes (chick peas, lentils or some kind of dried bean) or meat, seafood or chicken make easy options for a quick meal-in-a-dish. Lamb shanks and other slow-cooked meats are also good in soups and can be cooked ahead and frozen until ready for use. Freezing slows down any loss of nutrients and a frozen soup can be heated quickly for those occasions when you have little time.

CHICKEN SOUP – DOES IT HELP A COLD?

The TLC shown by someone making us chicken soup may lift our spirits and make us feel better even before we have eaten it. Inhaling the fragrant steam from a bowl of herby chicken soup can also raise the temperature of the airways and help loosen secretions. But chicken soup may do more. When fighting infections, our bodies produce white blood cells that also have inflammatory effects. Research shows that chicken soup contains anti-inflammatory compounds, released when chicken bones are boiled. Pulmonary specialists have shown that these compounds stop the white blood cells sticking together in the bronchial tubes where they cause swelling and excessive production of mucus. So it looks like the famous Jewish custom of serving home-made chicken soup to the sick has some scientific validity.

Spices
– add life to your food

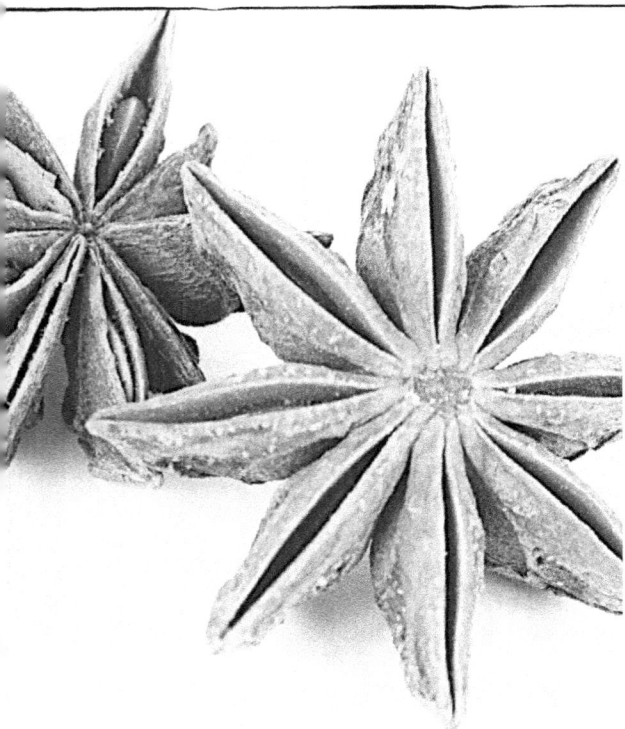

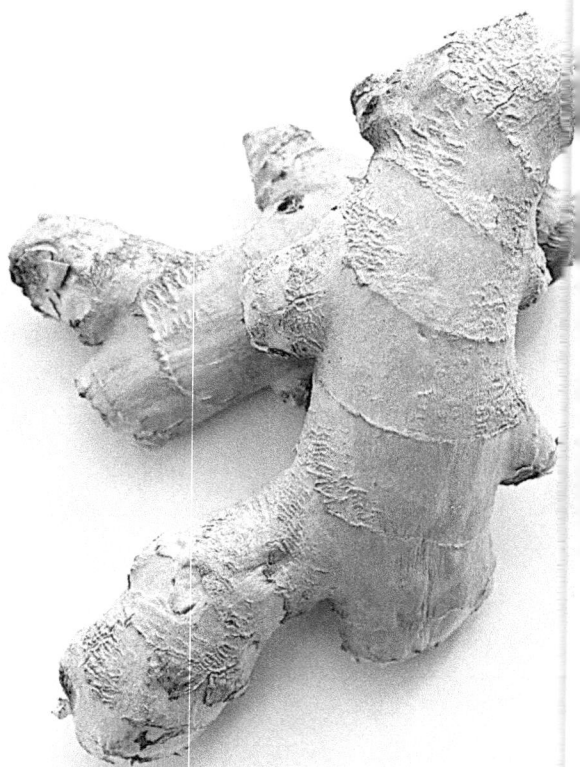

SPICES, FIRST BROUGHT TO EUROPE from India and then from the Spice Islands, have been important for thousands of years. From the fifteenth century onward, European nations competed for the highly profitable spice trade. Wars were fought, lives lost, and the triumphs of explorers such as Vasco da Gama, Christopher Columbus, Ferdinand Magellan and Sir Francis Drake were due to their search for exotic Eastern spices. Some spices have always been expensive and saffron still gets the prize for being the most expensive food per kilogram.

Spices add to the pleasures of many dishes. Fortunately, the days have long gone when spices were used to disguise foods that were no longer in prime condition. Many are high in minerals and dietary fibre, but in practice the small quantities consumed mean they do not make a significant contribution. On the other hand, their content of phytonutrients – mostly polyphenolic compounds – that may give protection against some common health problems is putting some of them into the spotlight.

Allspice

Sometimes called pimento, allspice is ground from the dried unripe berry of a species of myrtle tree that grows in the West Indies and Central America. The flavour is rather like a mixture of cinnamon, nutmeg and cloves and can be used in pickles, cakes, biscuits and some meat dishes. Oil pressed from allspice appears to have powerful antioxidant activity.

Anise

The Old World herb whose fruit produces aniseed, *Pimpinella anisum*, is used to flavour pastries, fish, meat and vegetable dishes as well as the liqueurs absinthe and pernod. Star anise is the dried fruit of an unrelated tree which grows in parts of Asia.

Asafoetida

A resin extracted from the plant *Ferula asafoetida* and ground into a powder. Used in Indian cooking, especially in fish dishes, asafoetida is reputed to alleviate gastrointestinal wind. It does this by causing small quantities of gas to join together, making a larger quantity which is easier to pass. The spice is also being investigated in laboratory studies for possible activity against cancer cells.

Caraway

The seeds of a plant that grows wild all over Europe and parts of Asia, raw or roasted caraway seeds were once a popular accompaniment to apples. Their main use today is in flavouring cakes, bread, cheese and cabbage dishes. Dental experts are currently researching the potential for a compound in caraway seeds to help prevent tooth decay.

Cardamom

Originally from India, cardamom seeds add a delicate flavour to pilaf and other rice dishes. Ground to a powder, cardamom is widely used in cakes and biscuits as well as in curries, pickles and chicken dishes. Cardamom-flavoured coffee is popular in Arab countries. The spice has widespread use in traditional medicine, and properties that may possibly stop blood cells sticking together and prevent the growth of cancer cells are currently being investigated.

Cassia

Taken from the bark of a tree of the laurel family that is native to Burma, cassia is also known as Chinese cinnamon. Its flavour is similar to cinnamon, but a little harsher and more suited to curries than sweets. The easiest way to distinguish the two is by colour: cinnamon is brown; cassia is a darker reddish brown.

Cinnamon

The dried inner bark of a tree belonging to the laurel family and native to Sri Lanka, cinnamon is widely grown in India, South America and the West Indies. Cinnamon was once valued more highly than gold and was the most valuable spice in the Dutch East India Company's trade. About 3000 BC, it played important roles in witchcraft, religious rites and embalming. Cinnamon is now used for flavouring baked goods, sweets, curries and drinks. Recent reports have shown that cinnamon stimulates the metabolism of glucose in rats. Human studies have given mixed results, possibly because it is difficult to consume a large enough quantity of cinnamon to cause any change in blood glucose levels.

Cloves

The small dried buds of a tree which originated in the Moluku (Spice) Islands in the East Indies, the name clove comes from the Latin word for 'nail', which the clove resembles. Historical records note that cloves have been used to sweeten the breath since about 300 BC. Most of the world's cloves are now grown in Tanzania and half the total crop is used in Indonesia, where cloves are mixed with tobacco. Oil of cloves contains eugenol, a substance with local anaesthetic properties that has been used for centuries to alleviate toothache. Cloves are used in cakes and other baked goods, and in pickles, chutneys and curries.

Coriander

Coriander (called cilantro in the United States) is used as both a herb (the leaves), and a spice (the ground seeds). Ancient Egyptian papyrus records show that coriander has been used for over 7000 years. It is popular in Thai cuisine, Indian curries and in some South American dishes.

Cumin

Sometimes spelled cummin. The seeds of this plant from the carrot family are widely used to flavour curries and various legume dishes in Asian cookery, breads and cakes in Europe and many dishes in South America (including chilli con carne). Iran produces most of the world's cumin powder. Cumin is rich in iron, containing 69 mg/100 g, so even 5 g could provide a significant proportion of the daily needs. The oil from cumin seeds is used in perfumes and as an ingredient in some liqueurs. The antioxidant content of the seeds is high but studies are needed to judge its effects on health.

Curry leaves

More correctly a herb than a spice, the leaves of the small tree *Murraya koenigii*, native to Asia and with a flavour similar to citrus, are dried and added to curries. Curry pastes and powders also contain ground curry leaves.

Curry powder

Ready-mixed curry powders contain many spices and may include cardamom, chilli, cinnamon, cloves, coriander, cumin, curry leaves, fennel seeds, fenugreek, garlic, ginger, mace, nutmeg, pepper, poppy seeds, saffron, tamarind and turmeric. The turmeric contributes the typical yellow colour. The flavour of curry powder decreases with time, so buy it fresh and in small quantities, or make your own by grinding your choice of spices in a mortar and pestle. Curry powder is rich in iron (almost 60 mg/100 g), so even a modest 5 g serve provides as much iron as a piece of red meat, although the iron from meat may be better absorbed.

Fennel seeds

The seeds of fennel are used in Asian and European cooking and have a slightly aniseed flavour. They are reputed to remove the smell of garlic from the breath. The seeds contain a chemical compound called estragole, which can be toxic in high quantities, and fennel teas should not be given to infants or children or used during pregnancy. The seeds are safe in culinary use, although allergic reactions occur in some people.

Fenugreek

A spice made from the slightly bitter mustard-coloured seeds of a small clover-like plant and usually included in curry powders. Due to their slightly 'raw' flavour, fenugreek seeds should be used sparingly, and may give the best flavour if they are lightly toasted before grinding.

Five-spice powder

A mixture of cinnamon, cloves, fennel seeds, star anise and peppercorns (preferably Szechuan pepper), used with chicken, seafood or meats, and popular in Chinese cuisine.

Galangal

This root spice is related to ginger, although its flavour is different and it lacks the 'bite' of its relative. Descriptions of the flavour of galangal include notes of earthiness, with pine or citrus characteristics. It is widely used in curries in Malaysia and Indonesia, in many Vietnamese dishes, and is also an ingredient in bitters and some liqueurs. In some countries it is known as lengkuas or laos. The root contains some potent compounds currently being researched for possible medicial use.

Garam masala

A mixture of aromatic spices used in Asian and Middle Eastern cooking. There is no set recipe, but the ingredients usually include cardamom, cinnamon, cumin, cloves, nutmeg and pepper. Unlike most spices, garam masala is added just before the end of cooking.

Ginger

The ground root of the ginger plant is used as a spice in both sweet and savoury dishes. The word ginger is derived from an old Sanskrit word meaning 'horn-shaped'. The underground stem of the ginger plant is a rhizome that shoots and forms roots. Ginger was first used as a food in China about 2500 years ago and is still widely used in Chinese and Japanese cooking, and has also found a place in Europe and North America. Studies show that ginger plays a powerful role in alleviating feelings of nausea. It is used for this purpose in nausea associated with pregnancy and some cancer treatments.

Juniper

Juniper berries are used in making gin but are also popular in dishes that include pork, veal and game meats. Juniper tea is used in some Scandinavian countries and is considered soothing. Note that some people develop allergies to juniper.

Mace

The outer covering layer of the nutmeg, mace comes from an ever-green tree native to the Maluku Islands of Indonesia. Mace is separated from nutmeg and allowed to dry before being cut into flakes or ground to a powder. Both mace and nutmeg were introduced to the Medi-terranean region by Arab traders some 800 years ago and generated a high income. The Dutch became most aggressive in their efforts to win the spice trade, destroying three-quarters of all the nutmeg trees to make the product a scarce and high-priced commodity. Mace has a slightly coarser flavour than nutmeg and is used in curries and pickles, rather than desserts.

Mixed spice

Usually a mixture of cinnamon, nutmeg and cloves, mixed spice is useful in both savoury and sweet dishes.

Mustard

Ground from the seeds of various types of mustard plant, mustard powder is mixed with water to release mustard oil. Depending on the type of seeds used, mustard may be pungently hot, spicy or mild. In general, French and German mustards tend to be blended with different herbs and vinegars and have a mild flavour. English, Chinese

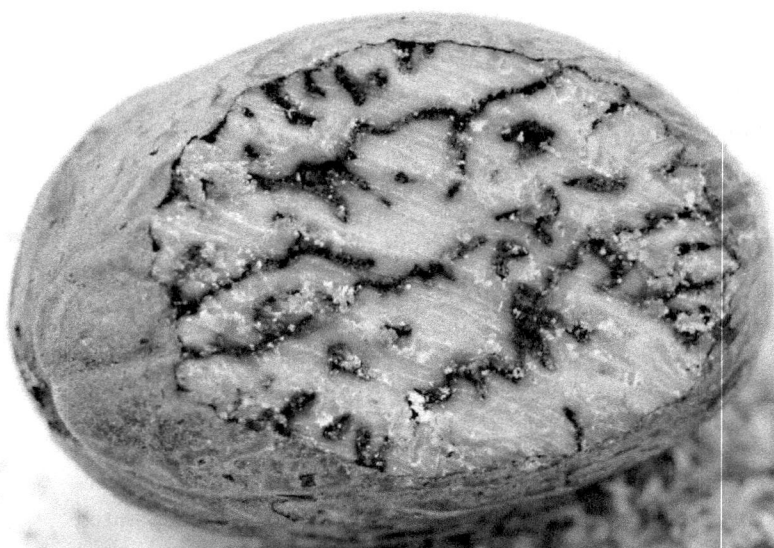

NUTMEG

and Japanese mustards are hotter. American mustards usually have added sugar and a mild flavour. Fine mustards from the Dijon region of France are made from de-husked mustard seed, although varieties containing whole seeds are also popular. Mustard is often added to vinaigrette dressings because the mustard oil acts as an emulsifier and helps bind and thicken the oil and vinegar. Mustard seeds are rich in omega 3 fatty acids, although the quantity consumed may be too small to have any measurable effect.

Nutmeg

The seed kernel of an evergreen tree which grows in the Maluku Islands (see Mace). Nutmeg is mainly used in small quantities in desserts, cakes, biscuits and curries. The oil in the nutmeg seed contains a toxic substance called myristin which acts as a strong hallucinogen, causing headaches, vomiting and stomach cramps. Such symptoms would only occur from consuming one or two whole nutmegs – which would be difficult, since nutmeg in large quantities is bitter.

Paprika

Made from powdered, dried sweet red pepper (capsicum), paprika is widely used in Eastern European cooking and provides a distinctive flavour to Hungarian goulash – and to many Spanish dishes. Paprika loses its flavour with storage.

Pepper

Both black and white pepper are the dried fruits of the tropical vine *Piper nigrum*, native to India, and are the most commonly used spices throughout the world. To make black pepper, the fruits are picked green, allowed to mature in the sun to produce a stronger flavour and then dried. For white pepper, the fruits are allowed to ripen to a red colour and are soaked in water, rubbed to remove the skins and dried. The sharp bite of pepper comes from an alkaloid called piperine. This substance can irritate the lining of the stomach.

Pink peppercorns, most of which come from plantations in Madagascar, are not true peppercorns but the dried berries of *Schinus molle*,

205

an evergreen tree native to South America and Mexico, and used in many countries as a shade tree and windbreak. The berries are cracked and used for flavour and colour. Some people experience an allergic reaction to pink peppercorns, but it is unclear whether this is due to the true pink peppercorn or a similar-looking product from the closely related tree *Schinus terebinthifolius*.

Szechuan (or Sichuan) pepper is also not a true pepper, but the seed pod of several species of prickly ash tree (genus *Zanthoxylon*) that grow in Szechuan in China. It has an aromatic flavour and can produce a slight tingle on the lips, but lacks any pepper-type heat. It is widely used in northern Chinese cuisine as well as in Japan and also Tibet and Bhutan, and is one of the few spices available in Himalayan regions. Ground Szechuan pepper is pale brown.

Tasmanian mountain pepper comes from the seeds of the pea-sized fruit of the *Tasmannia lanceolata* bush. Its 'bush food' flavour goes particularly well with kangaroo and emu but it is increasingly used in a wide range of dishes.

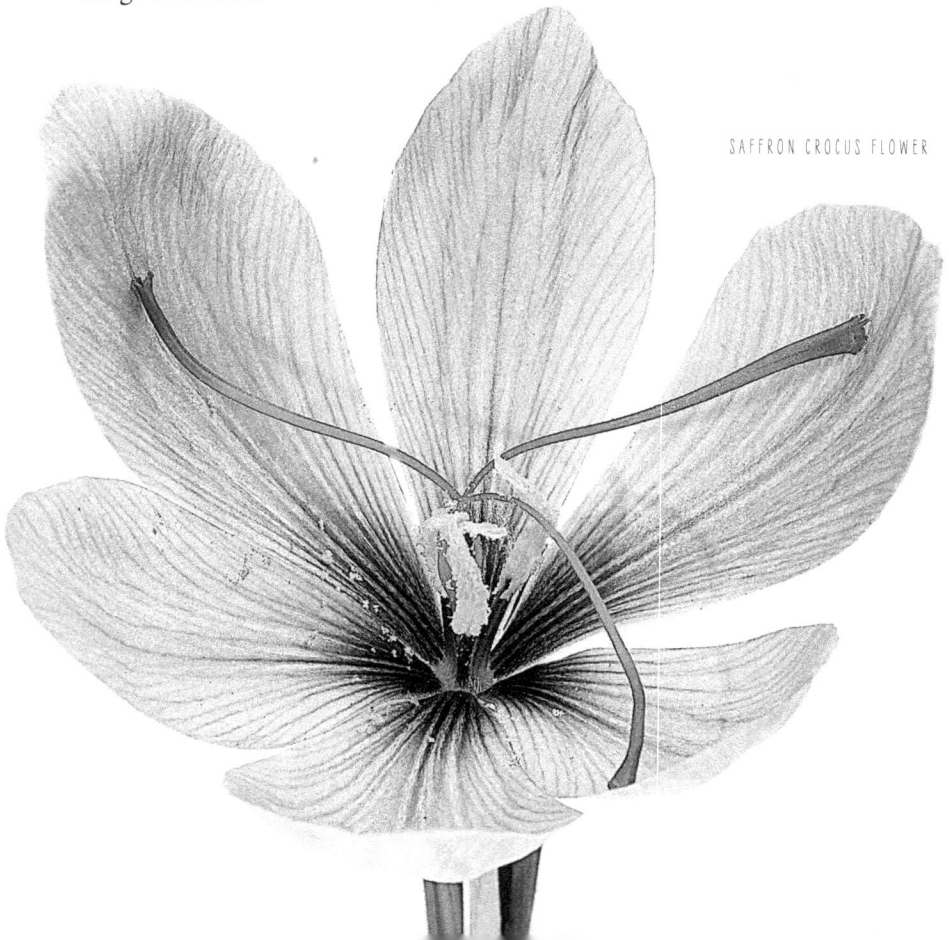

SAFFRON CROCUS FLOWER

Pimento

See Allspice.

Saffron

The dried stigma of the bulb *Crocus sativus*, saffron is the most expensive spice in the world. It must be harvested by hand, and over 1500 flowers are needed to produce 10 g of saffron. This valuable spice has been used for thousands of years and was introduced to Europe from Central Asia during the twelfth and thirteenth centuries. It is popular in Spanish and French cooking and has an important role in Indian and some Asian cuisines. Saffron is sometimes replaced with the cheaper yellow powder turmeric, but there is no comparison with the subtle and delightful flavour of the true saffron. Medicinal use of saffron has a long history.

Star anise

Star anise comes from the dried star-shaped fruit of a tree of the magnolia family, native to China. The pods are often used whole in cooking, but are not eaten. The seeds contained in the pod are ground to a powder that is rubbed into the skin of chicken or duck. The aniseed flavour comes from an oil which is similar to that found in anise. Star anise has been used for centuries in Chinese medicine, but toxic reactions have occurred in young children given a tea made with star anise.

Turmeric

The dried, ground stem of a plant found in Asia and the West Indies, turmeric is a bright yellow colour and is an ingredient of curry powders. It is also used as a fabric dye and has been used as a medical treatment in many parts of Asia for over 4000 years. Turmeric should be kept in a dark place since it loses its colour and flavour when exposed to sunlight. Studies shows that turmeric has anti-inflammatory, anti-microbial, anti-cancer and powerful antioxidant properties in the laboratory, but its absorption and uptake by cells is poor. Current research seeks to extract its valuable curcumin components and combine them in a complex compound that may be better absorbed.

Sugars
– are they really so sweet?

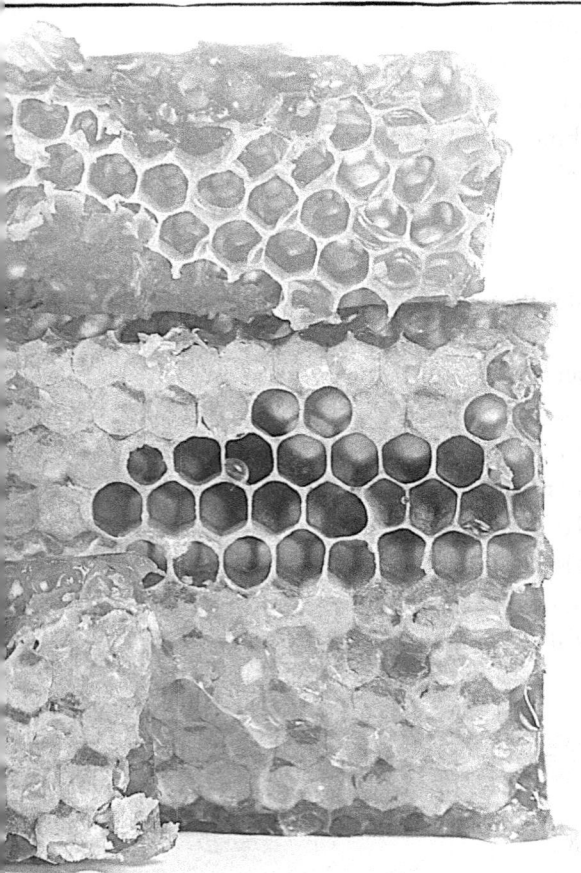

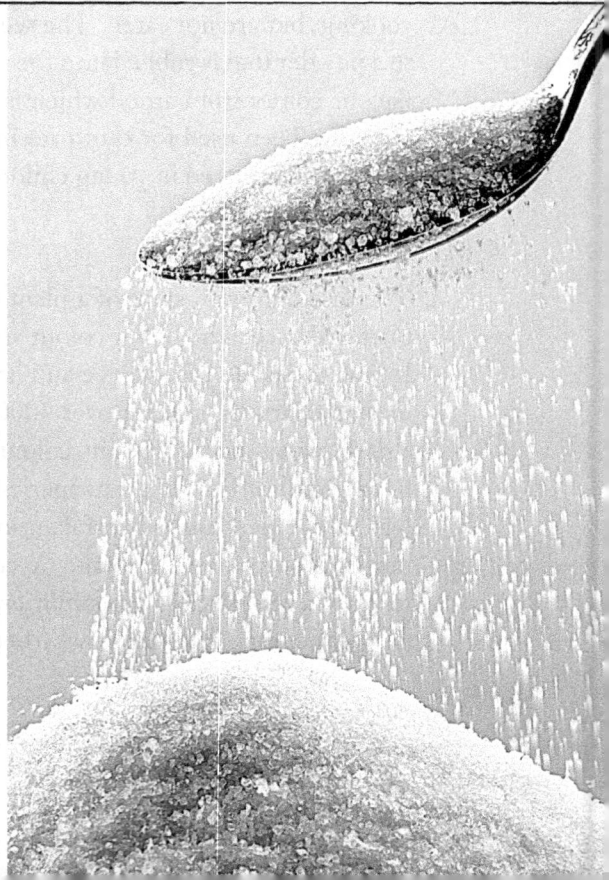

EVEN BEFORE THEY ARE BORN, the facial expressions of babies exposed to sweetness in their mother's amniotic fluid show pleasure, while they will purse their lips in response to anything bitter. The love affair with sweetness continues with the first taste of mother's milk and is confirmed when infants and children are comforted with something sweet to soothe life's little ills. The food industry reinforces the sweet deal through advertising and promotion of sweet foods and drinks. Millions of years ago, our ancestors probably also discovered that sweet foods tended to be safe to eat whereas bitter-flavoured plants were often poisonous. Sadly, our love of sugar and the push to get us to consume ever greater quantities by adding it to foods and drinks consumed at almost every meal means we now consume far more sugar that our sedentary bodies (and our teeth) can handle safely.

A bit about carbs

Carbohydrates consist of sugars and starches. The six main types of sugars found in foods can be classified as monosaccharides (one-sugar units) and disaccharides (two-sugar units). Starches are called polysaccharides and are made up of many glucose units.

The *monosaccharides* are:
- glucose (also called dextrose or grape sugar), found in fruits, vegetables and honey
- fructose (or fruit sugar), found in fruits, vegetables and honey
- galactose, mainly formed when milk sugar is digested.

Common *disaccharides* are:
- sucrose (ordinary table sugar), made up of one molecule of glucose and one of fructose
- lactose (milk sugar), made up of one molecule of glucose and one of galactose
- maltose (malt sugar), made up of two molecules of glucose.

Every gram of carbohydrate provides us with 17 kilojoules, the same as protein, but well below alcohol (29 kJ/g) and fat (37 kJ/g). The kilojoules from any kind of sugar can easily add up because consuming sugar doesn't necessarily make us feel full. A 375 mL can of soft drink has about 40 g (10 teaspoons) of sugar, but it does not make us feel any fuller than a can of artificially sweetened soft drink (which has no sugar) or the same volume of water.

209

Sources of sugar

Almost all sugar used in foods in Australia is sucrose from sugar cane, a natural mixture of 50 per cent glucose and 50 per cent fructose. In many European countries, sugar is extracted from sugar beet roots; this is also sucrose. In the United States, much of the sugar used in soft drinks and processed foods comes from corn syrup, which is a by-product of the corn grown and processed for animal feed. Corn syrup consists of a mixture of sucrose and fructose in variable proportions. The corn syrup used in soft drinks and most processed foods has 45 per cent glucose and 55 per cent fructose, which is only marginally different from the sugar from sugar cane. A high-fructose corn syrup (up to 90 per cent fructose) is used in confectionery. Corn syrup is not usually used in products made in Australia but may be present in confectionery imported from the United States.

Sugary foods

Many foods found in the supermarket are high in sugar, even when you might not expect it. For example, sugar is often the major ingredient (apart from water) in many sauces and marinades. Pre-sweetened breakfast cereals may contain up to 50 per cent sugar and even those bearing a Heart Foundation tick of approval may have over 30 per cent. Sugar is a major ingredient in confectionery, sweet biscuits, cakes, pastries and other desserts, ice cream, flavoured milk and yoghurt, jams, pickles and chutneys.

Why too much sugar can be a problem

DENTAL DECAY

Bacteria living in the plaque on the surfaces of teeth devour sugar, producing tooth-rotting acids in the process. The cost of filling the holes in

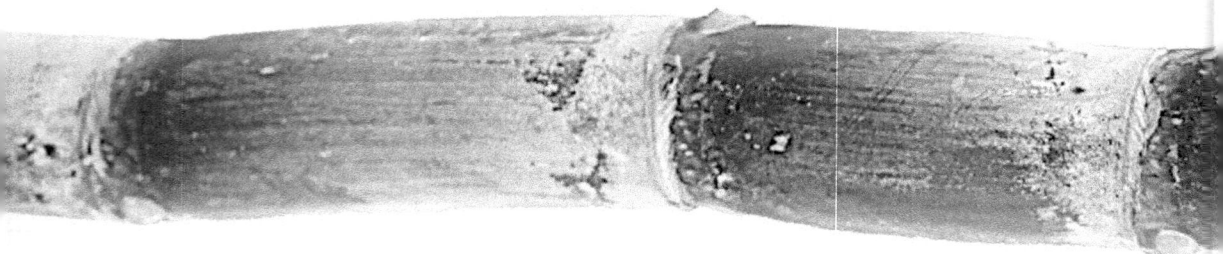

Australians' teeth is greater than all the costs associated with any other health problem, including heart disease or any type of cancer. Fluoride in water supplies and toothpaste cut dental decay, but cannot overcome the constant assault from constant snacking and the extra effect of acidic drinks (soft drinks, cordials, sports drinks, energy drinks, so-called 'vitamin waters' and fruit juice drinks). Tooth decay is on an upward trend, and although sugar isn't the only cause, it is a major factor.

OBESITY

Too many kilojoules from any source contribute to obesity. Fats have more than twice as many kilojoules as sugar, but it is sugar that makes the fats in cakes, pies, biscuits and desserts taste good. With the amount of sugar contained in so many foods and drinks, our overall intake is well above any level that can be accommodated by a largely sedentary population. Many studies now show that 'liquid' kilojoules from sugar-sweetened drinks are a particular cause of obesity because their low satiety (failure to make one feel 'full') does not curb intake of other sources of kilojoules. Those who need to lose excess body fat need fewer kilojoules, but no fewer nutrients, and thus it makes sense for would-be slimmers to make up the day's intake with foods that provide nutrients, while restricting those that provide kilojoules but few nutrients – such as fats, sugar and alcohol.

HEART DISEASE

New studies show that the more sugar consumed, the lower the blood levels of the 'good' HDL cholesterol that protects against heart disease. Sugar, and especially fructose (which some people wrongly think is a healthier sweetener), increases levels of fats known as triglycerides. Once the diet has more than 20 per cent of its energy from any kind of sugar (a common level in Australia), triglycerides rise. High triglyceride levels create another risk for heart disease.

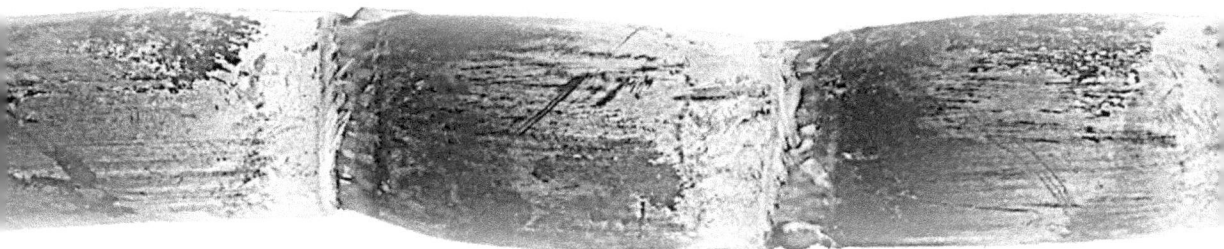

Sugar in the clear

HYPERACTIVITY

Claims that sugar causes hyperactivity in children have not been proved and research from the UK shows that it is more likely some of the colourings and preservatives present in sweet foods that lead to behaviour changes in some children.

DIABETES

Contrary to popular belief, sugar does not cause diabetes. An excess of kilojoules from any food leads to obesity – and it is obesity that is the greatest risk factor for type 2 diabetes. Sugar can easily supply excess kilojoules, but it is the surfeit of energy that is the problem rather than the sugar itself.

CANCER

The World Cancer Research Fund finds no convincing or probable evidence that sugar increases the risk of any type of cancer. These experts nonetheless urge caution with energy-dense foods and sugar-sweetened drinks because of their association with obesity and its link with some cancers.

Anything good about sugar?

Sugar tastes good – and the importance of pleasure from food should not be discounted. Small amounts of sugar do not appear to create damage within the body, so there is no need to avoid all sugar. Sugar may make some healthy foods more palatable. For example, most people enjoy a teaspoon of brown sugar or honey on top of rolled oat porridge. This amount is unlikely to be a problem, and is a better choice than eating a pre-sweetened cereal product where one-third of what you put in your breakfast bowl may be sugar. The kilojoules in sugar can also be valuable in survival situations, especially if combined with fat in a food such as chocolate.

How much sugar do we need?

We don't *need* to eat *any* refined sugar. We do need carbohydrates, but the natural sugars in fruit or milk or the starches in grains can supply these

212

along with a wide range of nutrients. The sugars we extract from sugar cane or sugar beet or even from fruit have no protein, vitamins, minerals, essential fats or dietary fibre – nothing, in fact that the body needs.

Even though we don't need refined sugar, small quantities are unlikely to be a problem. Recent data from the United States suggests a level of 5–10 per cent of energy from added sugars may be appropriate for their overweight population. The World Health Organization says that a generally healthy diet can accommodate up to 10 per cent of its kilojoules as sugar. For the average adult, that translates into 45–50 g of sugar a day. Many Australians consume twice as much. Children are particularly at risk since many choose sugary foods and drinks in preference to healthier options such as fruit or milk.

Sugar watch

The ingredients in foods must be listed in order of weight. To avoid disclosing that sugar may be the main ingredient in foods such as breakfast cereals and bars, three or more types of sugar may be used and listed. For example, an apricot bar that consisted of 60 per cent sugar and 40 per cent apricot could use 20 per cent each of three different sugars – and hence list apricot as the main ingredient. Look out for any of the following forms of sugar:

- sugar
- brown sugar
- raw sugar
- golden syrup
- treacle
- molasses
- maple syrup
- glucose
- dextrose (another form of glucose)
- glucose syrup
- sucrose (ordinary sugar)
- fructose (or fruit sugar)
- fruit juice concentrate (basically the nutrients are stripped away, leaving just fructose and glucose)
- maltose or malt sugar

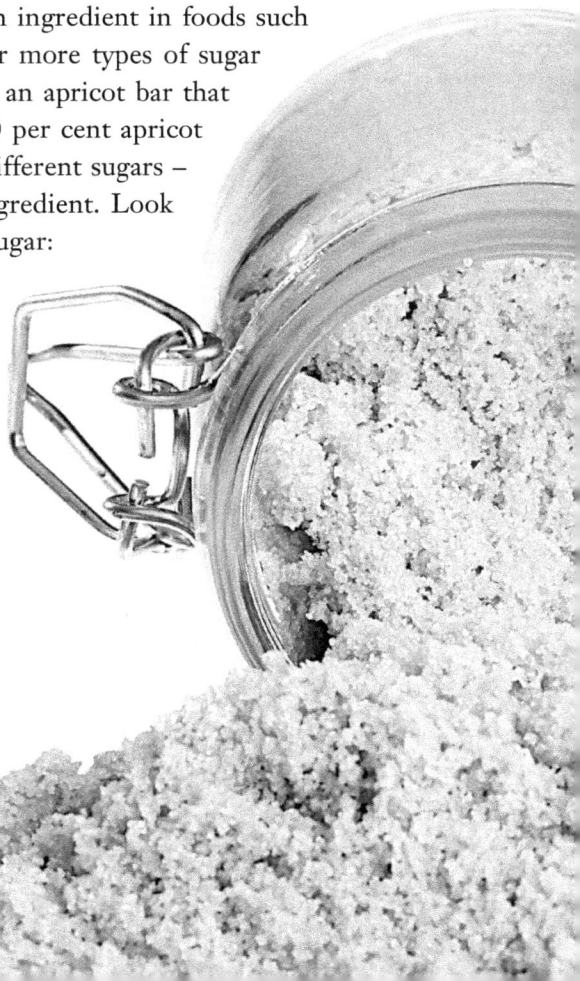

- corn syrup
- lactose
- sorbitol*
- mannitol*
- xylitol.*

Is fructose better?

Fruits contain a mixture of glucose and fructose, along with a collection of vitamins and minerals and dietary fibre. When fructose is extracted from fruit, the nutrients are left behind. Some people have promoted fructose as more desirable than sugar because it has a lower glycaemic index.** Others believe that fructose used as sugar may be more of a problem than sucrose from sugar cane because it is more easily converted into triglycerides. High levels of triglycerides are a problem for those with diabetes and can be one of the reasons leading to fat deposits in the liver (fatty liver). Research continues but experts believe that those who blame fructose for fatty liver and other health problems should blame a high intake of sugar-sweetened drinks – the major source of sugars (including fructose) consumed in the United States. Some Swiss research that claimed fructose leads to fatty liver gave participants an amount of fructose equivalent to drinking 4 L of soft drink a day on top of their normal diet. Repeat studies with the equivalent of 2 L of soft drink did not produce signs of fatty liver. Research is continuing to determine whether fructose has a specific ability to stimulate hunger and lead to overconsumption. In the meantime, it makes sense to reduce consumption of sugar, which will also reduce consumption of fructose. There is no need to avoid fruit.

*   Sugar alcohols – these contribute fewer kilojoules than sugar because they are not well absorbed. However, they cause diarrhoea and excessive amounts of wind.
** Glycaemic Index or GI measures how quickly the carbohydrate in a food is absorbed into the bloodstream compared with glucose. Glucose, which is absorbed very quickly, is assigned a value of 100; the lower the GI number the more slowly the substance is absorbed and the less likely it is that blood sugar levels will spike. Pure fructose has a GI of 23; pure sucrose has a GI ranging from 60–84. The actual GI of foods containing either of these sugars may be quite different from these values, however.

214

Tea

– green, black, white and herbal

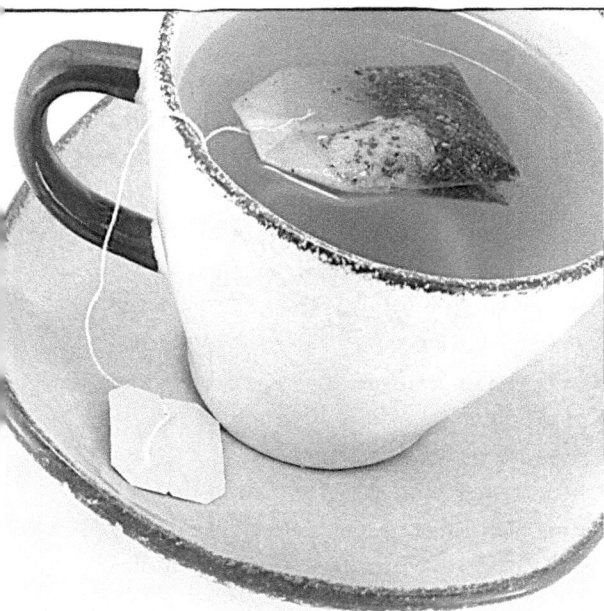

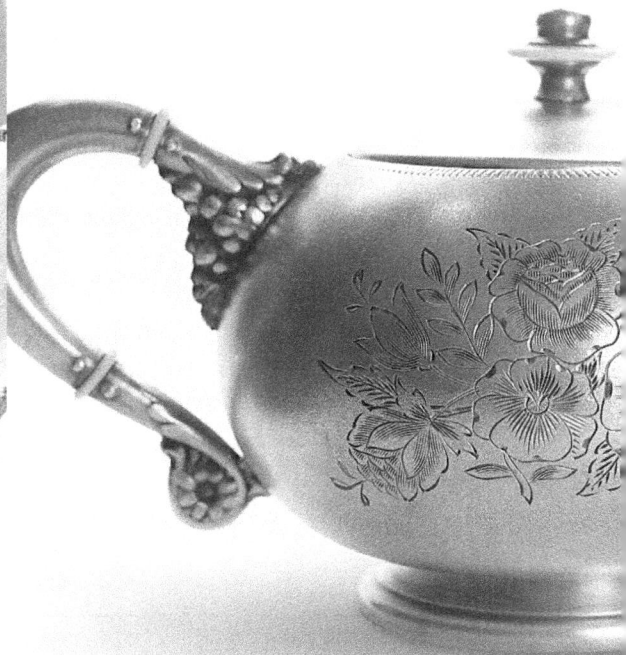

ON A WORLD SCALE, tea is the most popular drink after water, although in Australia it has been overtaken by coffee. All types of tea other than herbal teas come from *Camellia sinensis*, an evergreen shrub that prefers high regions or damp areas in the tropics and subtropics. Tea originated in India but was taken to China about 3000 years ago and became the national drink. The Dutch took tea to Europe in 1610, and some 30 years or so later it became common in England. Tea is now grown in China, India, Japan, throughout South-East Asia and in parts of Australia. In North Africa, a tea is made by infusing mint leaves, with or without tea leaves. The Nepalese add yak butter and salt to their tea while in the United States it is mostly consumed as sweetened iced tea. Its popularity is growing in many European countries.

Green, black or white?

The differences between various teas depend on climate, soil, freshness, the size of the leaf and flavour additives. About 2 kg of fresh leaves are required to make 500 g of dry tea. White, black and green tea all come from the same plant. White tea, the highest quality, comes from the flower bud and the top two leaves which enclose it. Black tea is made from fermented tea leaves; for green tea, the leaves are not fermented.

After harvesting, the leaves destined for green tea are heated with steam, then dried to prevent fermentation. For black tea, the leaves are torn and rolled by machine, then left at 27°C so that oxygen can help the natural enzymes in the leaves promote fermentation, turning the green leaves brown or black in the process. Fermentation is followed by 'firing', a process in which a current of hot air is passed over the leaves. The tea is then sorted into different grades by size of leaf, and broken leaf tea. It is often claimed that the larger the leaf, the better the quality of the tea. Others dispute this. Smaller leaves give stronger, darker teas. For tea bags, the leaves are cut by machine so that they will infuse more quickly into the liquid. The notion that the sweepings from the floor go into tea bags is a myth.

Oolong tea is a little different from either black or green tea in that the fermentation process is stopped at an early stage, giving a product midway between green and black tea in colour and flavour. It is also usually flavoured with jasmine flowers.

White tea includes the immature flower buds (which have fine whitish

216

hairs) and only very young tea leaves. In most brands, the buds and leaves for white tea are dried in sunlight and then steamed lightly and dried to prevent further fermentation. White tea has been used in China for centuries but its high price meant it was reserved for dignitaries. It is now sold throughout the world.

Various tea blends may contain a variety of herbs or flowers. Earl Grey tea is flavoured with the herb bergamot. Jasmine tea is a green tea blended with jasmine flowers. Some teas, such as Lapsang Souchong, have been exposed to smoke. Orange pekoe is a grade of tea rather than a flavour, and is made from the leaf bud and top two leaves of the leaf spray.

Tea and health

NUTRIENTS

Tea leaves contain fluoride, potassium, iron, niacin, protein and a range of minerals. When made into a drink, however, the quantity of tea used contributes very little of these nutrients, with the exception of fluoride. A cup of tea contains more fluoride from the tea leaves than from the water used to make it.

CAFFEINE AND TANNINS

Tea contains both caffeine and tannins. The caffeine content varies with the strength of the tea, but in general, average strength tea has about half the caffeine of brewed coffee. Weak tea has less caffeine. The tannins in tea are extracted from the leaves during infusion. The longer the leaves sit in the water, the greater the tannin content and the more astringent the tea. Tea poured quickly after being made has little tannin, but after five minutes brewing in the pot, the tannin content is much higher. Adding milk to a cup of tea binds the tannins and reduces their astringency.

For years, nutritionists have taught that tannins can interfere with the absorption of iron and therefore recommended that tea be drunk between meals. A new report has shown that, in practice, drinking tea with or straight after meals has no effect on iron absorption.

Green and black teas have a similar caffeine content, although it varies according to brewing time, and green tea is often brewed for a shorter time. Green and black teas contain different flavonoids, some of which function as antioxidants.

ANTIOXIDANTS

Different types of polyphenolic antioxidant compounds exist in green, black and white teas. Claims that one is superior to another usually arise because a researcher is looking only at the effects of one type of antioxidant. Recent research found that claims about antioxidants are also complicated by the fact that levels of antioxidants vary more than 10-fold in different samples of both green and white teas. Some white tea has more antioxidants than some types of green tea; other white teas have lower levels.

The antioxidants in green and white teas are a type of flavonoid called catechins. During the fermentation process to produce black tea, the catechins form polymers, which are classified into two major groups: theaflavins and thearubigins. Oolong tea contains smaller quantities of the flavonoids found in its green and black relatives. Whether the antioxidants in tea have any effects on health or preventing disease depends on how well they are absorbed by the body. This can differ in individuals as well as differing between teas.

CARDIOVASCULAR DISEASE, CANCER, BONE HEALTH, DENTAL HEALTH

Many studies show tea-drinking nations enjoy excellent cardiovascular health but it is difficult to know whether this is because the populations studied are usually not overweight and eat healthy diets. Is their longevity due to the tea or to other aspects of diet and lifestyle?

Some of the claims made for the health benefits of tea exaggerate research findings, often because sellers of tea assume that findings in laboratory tests (often using high doses of tea extracts) or with various animals apply to humans. Effects of the polyphenols in teas differ between animal species – with different results found even between rats and mice. The major problem involves the quantity of the potentially valuable compounds that are absorbed from the intestine. This varies with the individual and also with the particular tea.

Further studies are needed, but at this stage, studies into the effects of tea in humans show:

- good evidence of a reduction in cardiovascular disease in those who drink three or more cups of tea (green or black) a day
- evidence that black or green tea extracts may reduce the risk of some cancers in

some animals or in laboratory studies has not generally been backed in human trials, so it is not valid to make claims about green or black tea and the risk, incidence or treatment of cancers

- moderate evidence (but from only a small number of studies) that black tea may improve bone mineral density
- little evidence to support claims that tea reduces dental plaque, but the fact that tea is a source of fluoride deserves further study to see whether tea may protect against dental decay
- no evidence that green tea reduces the risk of type 2 diabetes
- no evidence that white tea helps prevent wrinkles
- no evidence that drinking tea helps reduce skin cancers
- no evidence of harm from drinking either green or black tea in moderate quantities.

WITH MILK?

Some studies claim that protective effects from tea are lost when milk is added. Others find no effect. Milk forms a complex with the catechins in tea, which is apparent in laboratory studies. However, recent research suggests these complexes are broken down during digestion, freeing the catechins. Most researchers now believe that adding milk to tea will have little practical effect on any potential benefits from its antioxidants.

HOW HOT?

Black tea is often sipped when it is very hot. This can damage the oesophagus, and higher rates of oesophageal cancer are found among people who drink very hot tea. In other words, there is absolutely no virtue in having a 'cast-iron' throat. Let your tea cool a little!

How much tea?

For most people, four cups of green, black or white tea a day is quite okay – more if the tea is weak.

Low-caffeine tea?

Some teas state that they are 97 per cent caffeine free. In fact, most teas contain no more than 3 per cent caffeine, so saying a tea is 97 per cent caffeine free has no special significance. Decaffeinated teas with no more than a negligible 0.3 per cent caffeine are available.

Herbal teas

These products are made from the leaves, roots, seeds or barks of various shrubs and trees. They have been used for centuries in many parts of the world. Today, herbal teas are used in place of regular tea or coffee, often by people who are trying to avoid caffeine or tannins. Some are used for their supposed health benefits.

Herbal teas are no more 'natural' than regular tea. Most do not contain caffeine, but many do contain tannins – sometimes more than regular tea. Uva ursi tea contains 15–20 per cent tannin, blackberry tea 14 per cent, peppermint has 3.5–12 per cent and lady's mantle 8 per cent.

There are no safety concerns about the fruit infusions and herbal teas generally sold in supermarkets. Chamomile tea, linden and redbush (rooibos) appear to be quite safe. Chamomile tea is reputed to have a mild calming effect, which may be due to its lack of caffeine. Tea made from hibiscus flowers is unlikely to do any harm in the quantities used and rosehip seems safe, although it does contain some tannins. Rosehip tea also has valuable pectins and vitamin C.

Some herbal teas may be hazardous to health. A few can have a stimulant action on the uterus and should not be used during pregnancy. These include juniper, mugwort, pennyroyal, raspberry, sage and yarrow teas. Other herbal teas contain alkaloids which can damage the liver and possibly lead to liver cancer. These include comfrey, larkspur and pennyroyal. Senna tea contains a potent drug which can cause diarrhoea and stomach cramps. Sassafras tea contains saffrole, once used as a food additive but now banned because it has been shown to cause liver cancer. Ginseng and liquorice root tea may increase blood pressure, while mistletoe can cause blood pressure to drop dangerously low.

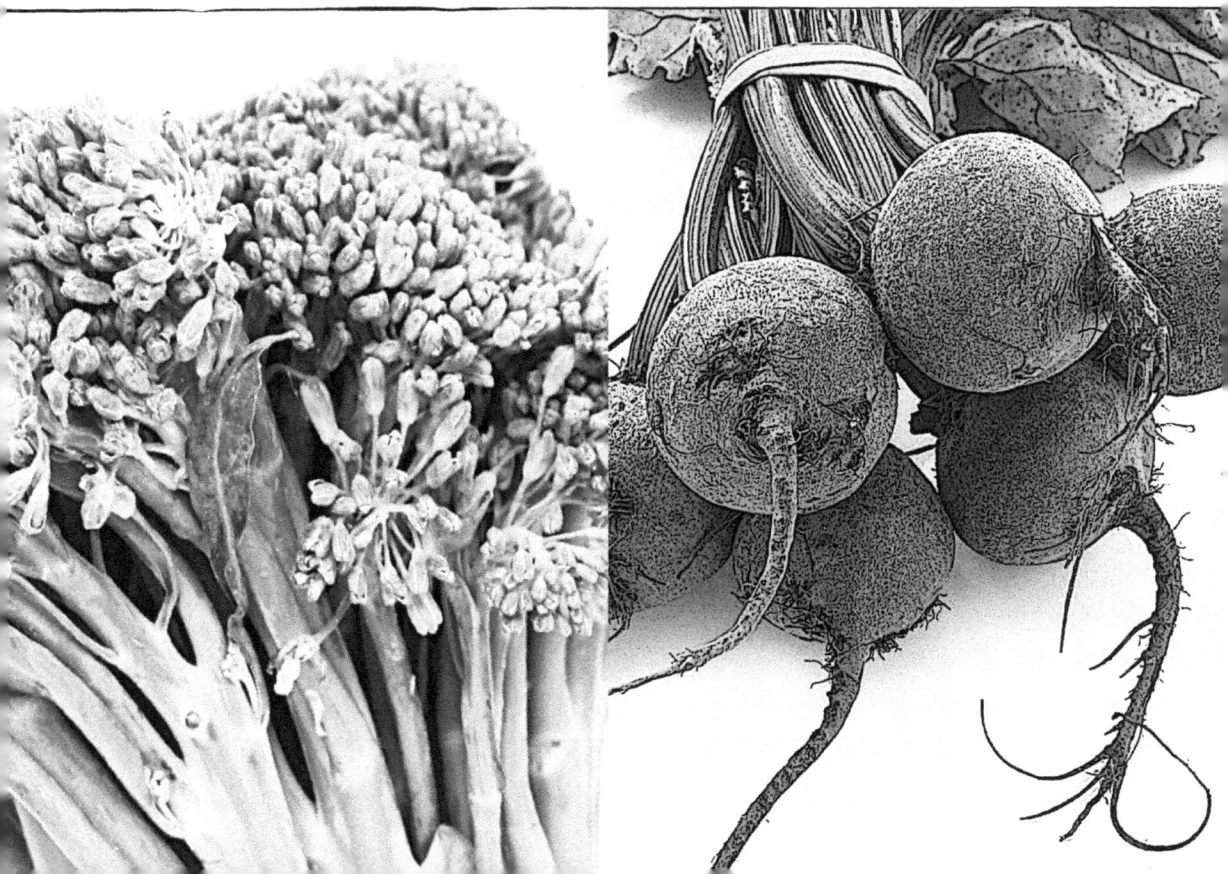

Vegetables

and herbs

NUTRITIONISTS ARE OFTEN ACCUSED of changing their minds, although major nutrition advice has hardly changed over the last 50 years. The call to consume more vegetables has always been with us, but the need has become more urgent as the evening meal is in decline, replaced by a series of snacks and fast foods.

Why we should eat them

There are two major reasons for eating vegetables: what they contain and what they don't contain. Their positive nutritional virtues include being a good source of vitamins (especially C, folate, E and beta carotene, which the body converts to vitamin A), minerals (especially potassium, magnesium, iron and zinc) and dietary fibre. Vegetables also contain literally hundreds of compounds classed as phytonutrients. These include a wide range of carotenoids and many compounds that have anti-cancer activity and contribute to eye health, especially in older people. The fact that vegetables have virtually no fat and contribute very few kilojoules is a bonus for an overweight population. No supplement can make up for a lack of vegetables.

Fresh vegetable juices contain the nutrients from vegetables, but miss out on fibre. Processed vegetable juices contain added salt, and even low-salt varieties still have much more sodium than straight vegetables.

How much?

Dietary guidelines recommend at least five servings of vegetables a day for adults and 2–4 servings for children. It sounds like a lot, but a serving is quite small – half a cup of cooked vegetables or 1 cup raw. A sauce for pasta might include onion, capsicum, mushrooms and tomatoes and provide 3–4 servings of vegetables. A green salad at the meal can add two more. Most people will need to include vegetables at two meals a day to get to five serves. For lunch, home-made vegetable soup in winter or a sandwich heaped with salad in summer can provide one or more servings. At the main meal of the day, vegetables should occupy half the plate.

222

Why we don't eat enough vegetables

In most parts of Asia, the Middle East and Africa, vegetables make a substantial contribution to meals. In Australia, few adults eat the recommended five servings a day and among children, 78 per cent of 4–8 year-olds and 95 per cent of 14–16 year-olds fail to meet the recommended 2–4 serves a day. Surveys show that most people know that vegetables are valuable and most adults intend to eat them, so it is not lack of knowledge or even intention. It appears that the major reason we don't meet our needs for vegetables is that dinner is often replaced by fast foods or frozen items such as pizza, or time commitments mean the evening meal is a snack. Those who eat in restaurants cite the fact that vegetables are no longer part of the meal and usually cost extra. Dislike of vegetables is a common reason for children not eating them.

The benefits of growing your own

At least six published studies show that where children attend a school that has a vegetable garden, or where vegetables are grown in the home garden, a child is much more likely to eat vegetables. And a child's acceptance of vegetables makes them much more likely to be served in the home.

Vegetables picked straight from the garden are convenient and almost always taste better. Children who see snow peas or carrots or cherry tomatoes or sweet corn or other vegetables growing in their own or a community garden are also more likely to try them and see them as a normal part of the meal.

Which vegetables come top of the class?

I would like a dollar for every time I've been asked which is the king of the vegetables. The answer is that it depends on what you are looking for. I can give you a list of vegetables according to their content of vitamin C or folate or dietary fibre or many other variables, but when we need a mix of hundreds of different compounds from vegetables, the only real answer is to include as many different types as possible.

Any vegetable is a good choice. To ensure a good balance of different nutrients, make choices from each of the following categories:

- *orange, red or deep yellow vegetables* such as pumpkin, carrots, kumara (orange-fleshed sweet potato), red capsicum, tomatoes, chillies, sweet corn
- *green vegetables,* such as broccoli, broccolini (a cross between broccoli and Chinese kale), green beans, peas, spinach, silverbeet (also known as Swiss chard), Asian greens, Brussels sprouts, watercress, green cabbage, Tuscan cabbage (a type of kale), lettuce, rocket, amaranth, asparagus
- *purple vegetables* such as red cabbage, beetroot, eggplant, purple onion
- *salad vegetables* such as one of the many types of lettuce, rocket, watercress, baby spinach, tomatoes, cucumbers, raw beetroot, capsicum, asparagus, snow peas, radicchio, curly endive, witlof
- *other vegetables* including cauliflower, potatoes, onions, spring onions, garlic, parsnips, zucchini, squash, mushrooms, okra, fennel, leek, kohl rabi, celery, celeriac, radish, swede, artichoke (Jerusalem or globe), water chestnut.

VITAMIN C

All vegetables provide this protective vitamin. Some have more than others, but choosing five serves a day will ensure an adequate supply. Top sources include capsicum, broccoli, Brussels sprouts, cabbage, Asian greens, broad beans, green beans, kohl rabi, spinach, watercress and chillies. Potatoes are a valuable source of vitamin C. Steam them in their jackets to prevent the vitamin escaping.

DIETARY FIBRE

All vegetables provide dietary fibre, both soluble and insoluble. The best sources include peas, broad beans, Brussels sprouts, broccoli, cauliflower, sweet corn, spinach and fennel.

CAROTENOIDS

Taking its name from carrots, beta carotene, which the body converts to vitamin A, is found in all orange and green vegetables. In green vegetables the beta carotene is masked by chlorophyll pigments. Various brightly coloured vegetables also have particular types of carotenoids that are valuable: tomatoes are rich in lycopene, a carotenoid that may give protection against prostate cancer; spinach is an excellent source of two carotenoids called lutein and zeaxanthin that are important for eye health.

FOLATE

This B complex vitamin is found in many leafy greens (its name comes from *folium*, Latin for 'leaf'). Top sources include Asian greens (especially flowering cabbage and mustard cabbage), spinach, broccoli, watercress, endive, asparagus, beetroot, cauliflower and sweet corn.

CARBOHYDRATE

Most vegetables contain very little carbohydrate. Diets that list vegetables as having a low glycaemic index (GI) are confusing. The GI measures how rapidly a portion of food containing 25 or 50 g of carbohydrate is converted to blood glucose; the lower the GI, the slower the conversion rate. Most vegetables have less than 1 g of carbohydrate per 100 g, and so they do not have a GI. Potatoes, sweet corn, green peas, cassava, sweet potato and taro are the main vegetables that supply some carbohydrate. Sweet corn, green peas and some types of sweet potato have a low GI.

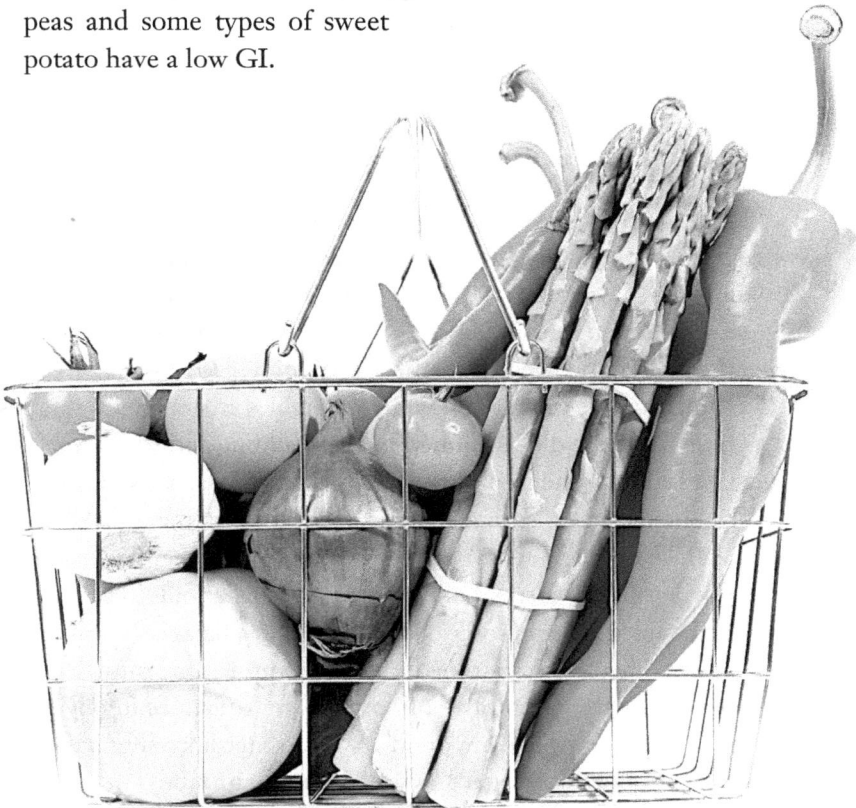

225

The floury kind of potatoes that mash easily have a high GI whereas those with a more waxy texture (which don't mash well) have a moderate GI. This is of little consequence since protein sources such as meat, fish or chicken will slow down the rate of digestion. People with diabetes should avoid a meal consisting solely of high GI potatoes – but that would be an unbalanced meal for anyone. Cutting out potatoes because of their GI is not justified. Cutting down on chips, potatoes baked in any kind of fat, and potatoes mashed with cream and butter may be wise for everyone.

ANTI-CANCER COMPOUNDS

Research is continuing but so far, researchers have identified anti-cancer compounds in:

- vegetables of the *Brassica* genus, including broccoli, Brussels sprouts, cabbage, cauliflower, kohlrabi and rocket
- vegetables of the *Allium* genus, including onions, garlic, spring onions, eschallots
- *purple-coloured* vegetables such as eggplant and red cabbage that contain pigments called anthocyanins.

Cooked or raw?

Cooking causes losses of some vitamins but makes other compounds more available. Vitamin C, folate and thiamin (vitamin B1) are lost during cooking, to a lesser degree with microwaving or steaming and a larger degree with boiling. Roasted vegetables retain more vitamins than boiled vegetables, and stir-fried vegetables even more. Overcooked vegetables suffer much greater losses. Soaking vegetables in water also causes loss of vitamins and the old-fashioned habit of adding bicarbonate of soda to greens to brighten their colour causes extensive loss. Don't do it.

Carotenoids are absorbed better from cooked than raw vegetables. However, we do not need to eat everything cooked; carrots, for example, still contribute very worthwhile quantities of carotenoids in their raw state. Some vegetables raw and some cooked provides a balance. Carotenoids are also absorbed better when some fat is eaten at the same meal. So adding a dressing with extra virgin olive oil, or cooking tomatoes in olive oil helps us absorb these valuable compounds. We can therefore shun fat-free salad dressings on valid nutritional – as well as taste – grounds.

Potatoes – are they fattening?

It is difficult to ever get fat on vegetables, and that applies to potatoes, since they are one of the most filling foods and few people can eat enough of them to overdo their kilojoule needs. The problem with potatoes is that their starchy carbohydrate soaks up fat, whether it is oil used for chips or roast potatoes, or butter, margarine or any kind of cream mashed into them or served with them. The added fat usually provides more kilojoules than the potato. Small new potatoes steamed in their skins and tossed with a little extra virgin olive oil and fresh herbs are delicious hot or cold.

How to encourage children to eat their vegies

As mentioned previously, the best way to encourage children to eat vegetables is for them to grow them. Snow peas, lettuce, cherry tomatoes and English spinach can be grown in pots on a balcony. Many children and some adults do not like strong-tasting vegetables such as silverbeet, broccoli and Brussels sprouts. (Researchers have dubbed children like this 'super-tasters', since their keen palate can identify even a tiny portion of some vegetables.) Children can get used to these vegetables, but it may take time. In some studies, children had to taste a vegetable an average of eight times before they would accept it. The idea is to tell the child they do not have to eat all of the vegetable, but they must take one bite. Gradually their tastebuds get used to the flavour.

Teaching children to cook also helps them accept vegetables. When primary schools have a kitchen garden and the children cook what they have grown, sitting down to eat with their classmates and teacher, they accept vegetables. In one study in Melbourne, the whole family ate more vegetables when a child attended a school with a kitchen garden program.

Grated vegetables like carrot and zucchini can also be incorporated into various dishes such as hamburger patties and pasta sauces, although I don't like trying to hide them in this way. Stir fries are popular with a lot of children, and many are also quite happy to eat raw vegetables.

A platter of red, green and yellow capsicum strips, snow peas, cherry tomatoes, green beans, carrot sticks and raw or lightly steamed asparagus (or just three or four of these) is usually popular, especially if served with an avocado dip, natural yoghurt, beetroot dip (puree beetroot with yoghurt and a spoonful of tahini) or pesto.

Herbs

Herbs are generally rich in nutrients, but we usually don't eat enough for them to make much nutritional contribution. There are exceptions to this. For example, tabbouli uses a lot of parsley, home-made pesto incorporates enough basil to add nutrients, and some Middle Eastern recipes use whole bunches of mint or parsley or coriander.

Parsley is particularly rich in iron, calcium, potassium, vitamin C and folate, and beta carotene. Adding a bunch to a recipe makes a significant contribution to all these nutrients, whereas a sprig used as a garnish just looks pretty.

We use rosemary only in small quantities, but it contains several acids, including carnosic acid and rosmarinic acid, that may have anti-cancer activity. Researchers are identifying more potent and potentially beneficial anti-cancer compounds in other fresh herbs.

A few herbs are actually dangerous and should not be eaten. They include pennyroyal, which can damage the liver and is especially hazardous during pregnancy. Hyssop should be avoided during pregnancy. An emergency poultice made from comfrey can be applied to unbroken skin around a broken limb but the herb is not suitable for internal use because it contains alkaloids that can damage the liver and could lead to liver cancer. Claims that comfrey contains vitamin B12 are false. The compound it contains is an analogue of vitamin B12 that cannot be absorbed or used by humans.

Water
– essential to life

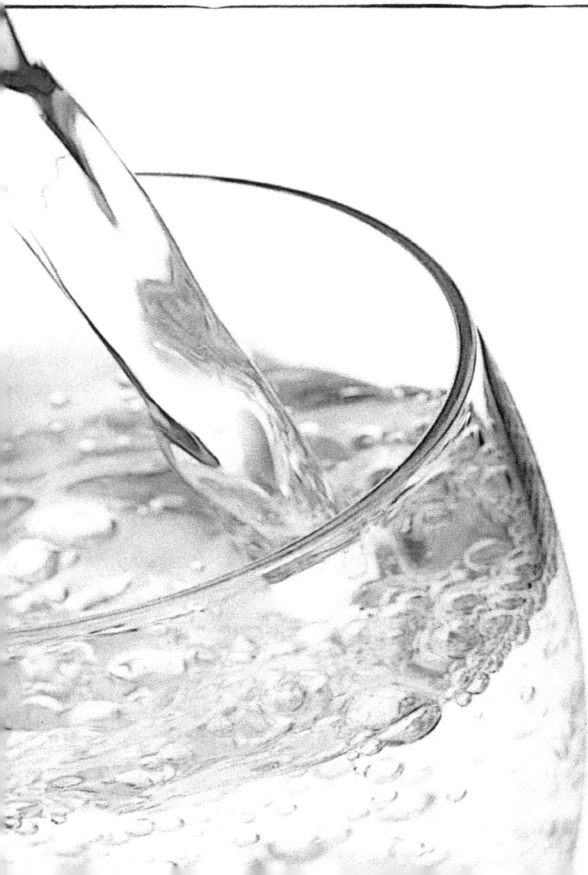

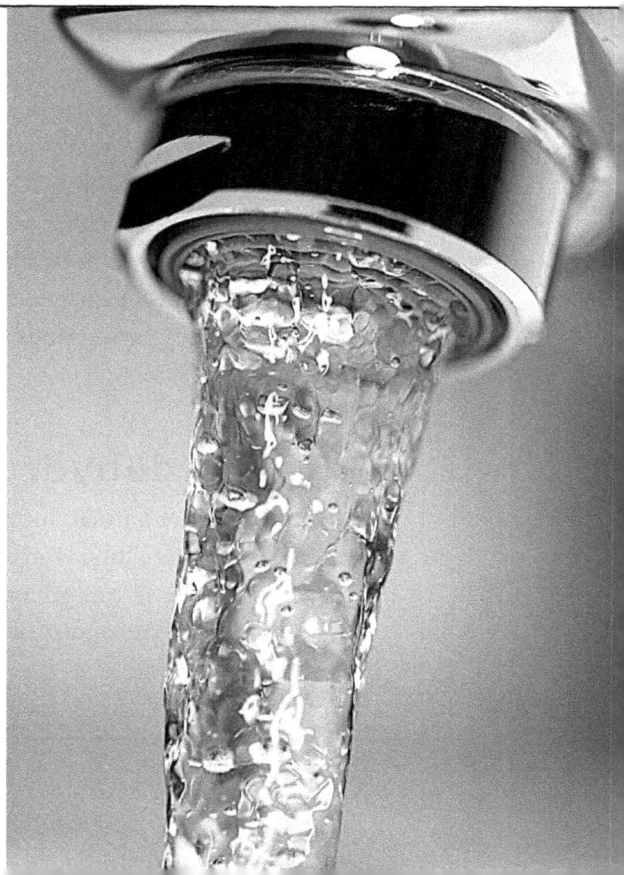

THE UBIQUITOUS BOTTLE OF WATER has become a seemingly indispensable accessory. Some people apparently can't get through a meeting, bus ride, lecture, church service or a short wait at the doctor's surgery without frequent sips of water. Some swimmers at my local pool even stop every two laps to take a few sips 'to prevent dehydration'.

Why we need water

Water is more important to life than food. We can survive only a few days without it. Every cell and organ in the body needs water to function. Water is the solvent for the body's chemical reactions, it transports nutrients, removes waste products, acts as a lubricant and maintains body temperature through sweating.

Around 55 to 70 per cent of the body's weight is made up of water. As well as making up the basis of blood and digestive juices, water is a vital component of lean muscle tissue and bones. The leaner you are, the higher your percentage of water – disproving the common claim that those who are overweight have 'fluid retention'.

The body's water content can fluctuate safely to some extent, but a drop of 4 per cent (equivalent to approximately 2.5 per cent of body weight) will substantially impair physical performance and lower efficiency. A loss of 5 to 10 per cent of the body's water (equivalent to 3 to 6 per cent of body weight) produces fatigue, mental confusion and apathy. If more than 15 to 20 per cent of the body's water is lost, death results. On the other hand, overzealous use of water can also be hazardous, as has been seen in deaths among a small number of athletes who have drunk excessive quantities of water and suffered water intoxication and hyponatraemia (a serious and potentially fatal dilution of the body's electrolytes).

Thirst and dehydration

Like every other animal, humans have evolved to instinctively quench thirst with water. Thirst is an excellent indicator of fluid needs, although the thirst response can go awry in the frail aged, and young children may not always recognise when they are thirsty. During strenuous physical activity, the thirst response can be slow to respond and athletes engaging in prolonged activity may need to drink a little more than their thirst dictates. Under normal circumstances, however, the idea that feeling thirsty means you're already dehydrated is an attempt to medicalise a normal bodily function. It is equivalent to saying that feeling hungry means you are already malnourished. Thirst is simply the body's inbuilt method of telling us to have a drink, just as hunger tells us we need food.

The idea that 'thirst = dehydration' has been pushed by some companies marketing bottled water or other drinks for 'rehydration'. The notion has sold a lot of bottled water, sports drinks, energy drinks, soft drinks and sugary waters with added vitamins, but it should be seen largely as marketing hype. Unless there is some relevant medical situation as may occur with some elderly people, infants and others with vomiting or diarrhoea, diuretic medications, kidney stones or some other medical conditions, thirst is a reliable indicator of fluid needs.

Eight glasses a day?

Professor Heinz Valtin, the author of several textbooks on kidney function, looked into the origins of the recommendation to drink eight glasses of water a day. Valtin thinks the idea may have originated from the Food and Nutrition Board of the National Research Council in the United States, which in 1945 recommended 1 mL water for each calorie of food consumed. Since the average person needs about 2000 Calories (8400 kJ) a day, this equates to 2000 mL – or eight glasses of water. However, the same Nutrition Board also stated that 'most of this quantity is contained in prepared foods'. Professor Valtin says that no studies support the idea of eight glasses of water for everyone, and disputes the notion that it is necessarily correct under normal conditions.

For a small sedentary person in a moderate climate eight glasses may be too much, whereas someone who is large or is engaged in strenuous physical activity, exposed to very hot conditions, or taking a long flight, will need much more.

Can drinks containing caffeine be 'counted' as fluid?

There is no reason why tea and coffee cannot be counted towards fluid requirements. It is a myth that these beverages lead to dehydration. Both contribute fluid, and even though they may provoke a mild diuresis the passage of fluid through the kidneys is one of the reasons we need fluids.

Does drinking water improve concentration?

True dehydration does have adverse effects on concentration, but there is no evidence that most people are dehydrated. Extra water would only be required between normal break periods in hot climates.

Does drinking water prevent over-eating, flush out fat or boost metabolic rate?

There is no evidence to support any of these claims. If they were true, it is unlikely that the average Australian would be overweight or obese.

Will water prevent constipation and does 'flushing' the colon prevent bowel cancer?

Constipation is a common problem in Australia. The best way to combat simple constipation is to increase the intake of foods that provide dietary fibre. People who are genuinely dehydrated are likely to be constipated, but studies where fluids have been increased have not shown any benefits for stool frequency or consistency in children or adults. Flushing the colon, from either end of the intestine, will not prevent bowel cancer.

Is water a tonic for the skin?

Healthy skin requires adequate water – just like every other organ in the body. Dehydration can be diagnosed by skin that is so dry that it does not shrink back when lightly pinched. Drinking water is a healthy habit, but consuming water beyond satisfying normal thirst has no special benefits for the skin.

Bottled water

Less than 20 years ago, annual world consumption of bottled water was approximately 2 billion litres. By 2007, this had increased to 206 billion litres – most of it sold in countries with an adequate, safe water supply. Australians' annual bottled water consumption is approximately 242 million litres. This has put a slight dint in the sales of juices and sweetened soft drinks, but overall sales of sweetened drinks continue to rise. Bottled water represents extra sales.

Those who buy bottled water may be willing to pay for it although, somewhat ironically, those who could benefit from bottled water because of unsafe water supplies can't afford it. Bottled water has the edge over soft drinks because it has no kilojoules and no added sugar or other additives, but tap water makes even more sense, especially for environmental reasons. New designs in water fountains also make clean tap water a public possibility.

Bundanoon, a small town in the Southern Highlands of New South Wales, made headlines when local shopkeepers decided to stop selling bottled water. A commercial company wanted to take water from a local spring, truck it over a long distance to a bottling plant and cart it back to sell to the townsfolk and visiting tourists. The shopkeepers called a public meeting and received overwhelming support to install water fountains so that people could fill their own bottles with Bundanoon's fresh – and delicious – water, free of charge. The move has also reduced the litter problem from discarded bottles.

Some designer waters sold in high-priced restaurants cost up to 10 000 times the price of tap water. A more modest $2.50 for a 600 mL bottle of water is still over 5000 times the cost of getting it from the tap. Consider too that although some bottled water may come from a spring, much of it is simply filtered tap water. Tests of bottled waters also show that some may carry more bacteria than the safe tap water available in most parts of Australia.

The price paid for bottled water does not include the costs associated with environmental damage. Production, transportation, storage and refrigeration of bottled water create a massive carbon footprint. The billions of bottles sold each year involve greenhouse gas emissions from their production, collection, recycling and disposal. Even though the industry has moved to lighter weight bottles, over 300 000 barrels of oil are required for Australia's yearly usage of polyethylene terephthalate (PET) bottles. The manufacture of every tonne of PET produces three tonnes of carbon dioxide. PET bottles can be recycled, but 65 per cent of them are not – and in Australia over 76 000 tonnes end up as litter, making up 38 per cent of all roadside rubbish. Bottled water may be a marketing success, but it is an ecological disaster.

Wine

– and other alcoholic drinks

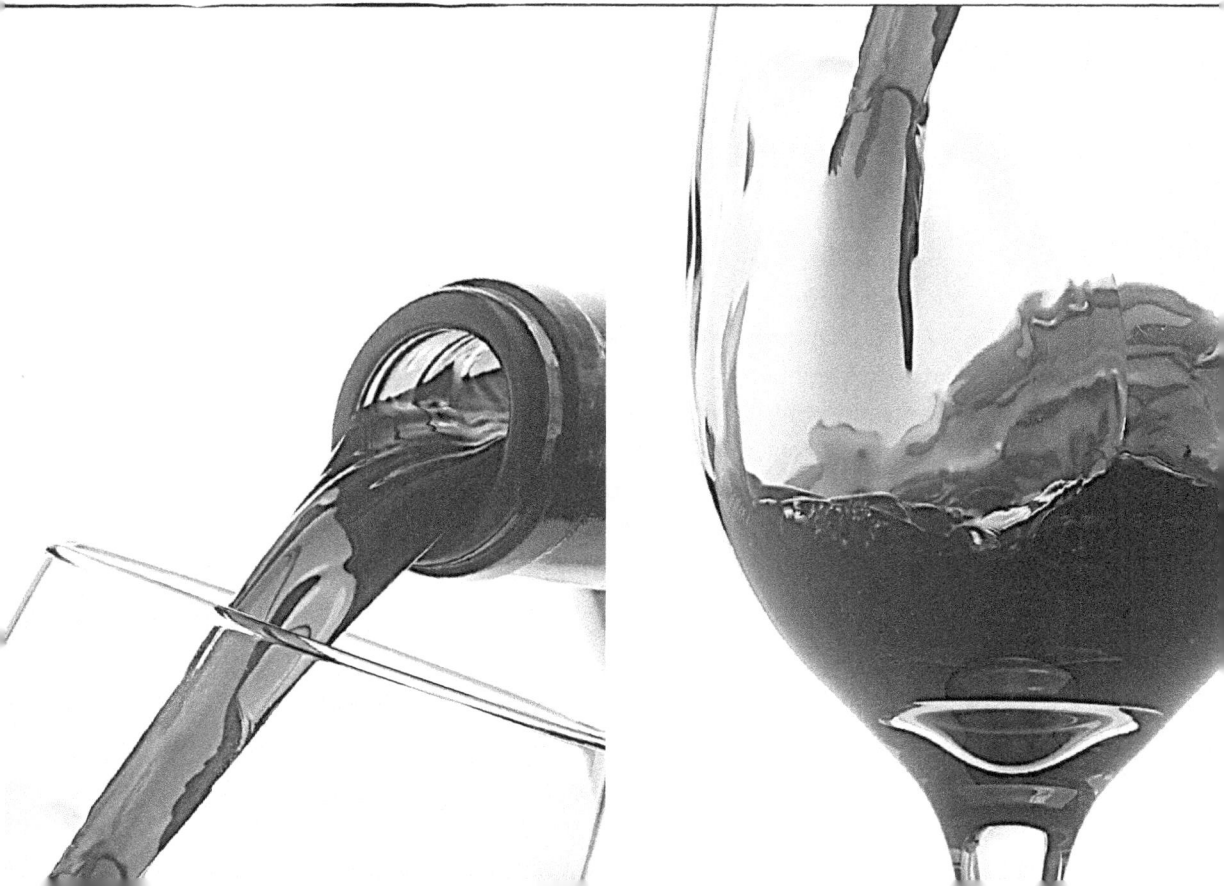

NO ONE NEEDS ALCOHOL, but civilisations throughout history have found ways to ferment sugars in plants to produce alcohol, which they have used as a food and a drug. In small quantities, alcohol has some overall benefits and red wine has some specific plusses. However, with alcohol, more is *never* better, and that applies to every kind of alcoholic beverage.

The fate of alcohol in the body

Alcohol is absorbed from the stomach as well as the small intestine. About 20 per cent of alcohol consumed is absorbed directly into the bloodstream from the stomach. This level may be higher if you drink on an empty stomach and the effect is especially rapid with anything fizzy such as Champagne, whisky with soda, or gin and tonic. The remaining 80 per cent is absorbed from the small intestine. Once alcohol passes into the bloodstream, it is rapidly distributed throughout the body and produces a range of effects. A small concentration of alcohol in the blood produces a feeling of relaxation as some of the usual inhibitions are released.

Alcohol is processed by the liver at a rate of about 7 g an hour. A 'standard drink' has about 10 g of alcohol. Trying to speed up the rate at which alcohol is metabolised by the liver is futile. Exercise, coffee, energy drinks and vitamins have no effect. Taking a large quantity of fructose may hasten the removal of alcohol, but the quantity needed produces nausea and vomiting. The only way to remove alcohol from the body is to wait until the liver processes it.

Each gram of alcohol contributes 29 kJ, much more than the 17 kJ/g from proteins or carbohydrates, but less than the 37 kJ/g from fats. Beer contains a small amount of carbohydrate, but the quantity contributes only a small percentage of its kilojoules. The assumption that low-carb beer is useful for weight control ignores the fact that the major factor of relevance is the alcohol content. Most low-carb beers have a similar alcohol level to regular beer. Light (low-alcohol) beer is a healthier choice. The only wines that contribute a significant quantity of carbohydrate along with their alcohol content are sweet dessert wines.

236

Any benefits?

Benefits from alcohol only occur with a low intake and are reversed when intake increases. Potential benefits are largely seen in those over 45 years of age, and the risks outweigh any benefits in people younger than 45. None of the benefits is enough to justify non-drinkers changing their ways. Benefits include:

- Alcohol increases 'good' HDL cholesterol. This is a function of the alcohol itself, and is not confined to the consumption of red wine, as is popularly believed.
- Some types of alcohol cause the body to make fewer of its normal clotting proteins. This may be a reason why red wine gives some protection against the formation of blood clots.
- More than 200 compounds that can act as antioxidants are found in alcoholic drinks. Red wines made from thick-skinned grapes such as cabernet sauvignon have particularly high levels of these potentially protective substances. Much of the current research has focused on a polyphenol called resveratrol that has some anti-inflammatory properties and may also contribute to reducing the incidence of heart disease. Resveratrol is also found in peanuts as well as fresh grapes, but some studies show that fermentation increases its potency.
- Drinking a *small* amount of alcohol may also have some social benefits. One recent study of healthy Japanese and British men identified a strong connection between moderate social drinking and reduced incidence of heart disease. After a drink or two (but not more), the men showed a reduced level of what researchers call 'vital exhaustion', a mental state related to hostility and burn-out. This and other studies on such associations show a J-shaped curve where the risk falls with low alcohol consumption but rises sharply for higher consumption. The effects are independent of the type of alcoholic beverage consumed.

Harmful effects

There are whole books on the harmful effects of alcohol. Too much alcohol from any type of drink increases the risk of high blood pressure, heart disease, stroke, dementia, liver disease, several common cancers, pancreatic problems and depression. More than one drink a day markedly increases the risk of breast cancer, especially in those women who have a low intake of foods high in folate (vegetables, whole grains, legumes).

237

Those who drink heavily also suffer impairment of their immune system, with higher risk of infections, poor wound healing and prolonged recovery from trauma. Alcohol can also trigger a cascade of problems due to its effects on the central nervous system. The effects begin at the frontal lobe and move into the areas of the brain that control speech, vision and the coordination of muscles. This eventually causes poor coordination and behavioural changes that stem from inability to reason and impaired judgement, and can lead to domestic violence, aggression, traffic accidents and injuries, loss of productivity at work, memory loss and many criminal activities.

The old idea that alcohol is warming is incorrect; it does cause flushing of the skin, but this is followed by a loss of body heat to the air. It is therefore foolish to give alcohol to anyone who is suffering from exposure or any type of stress.

THE 'BEER GUT'

Alcohol is not directly converted to fat, but that doesn't mean drinkers don't get fat. The body burns the kilojoules from alcohol before it uses up those from carbohydrates, fats or proteins – and while it is busy burning off the grog, what we eat easily ends up as fat. The combination of beer and chips, crisps, sausages and other fatty meats is particularly problematic. Beer and salad would be safer! Some people think a beer gut is due to an enlarged stomach that stretches from holding large quantities of beer. In fact, a beer gut is more correctly called a 'fat gut'. The excess fat settles around vital organs and correlates with fat around the waist and on the upper body.

PREGNANCY AND BREASTFEEDING

Alcohol crosses the placenta. Large amounts consumed during pregnancy result in foetal alcohol syndrome and permanent problems for the child throughout life. Even moderate drinking during pregnancy can have adverse effects on the baby's brain. A single alcoholic drink is unlikely to cause obvious damage but, since doctors cannot be sure that no damage occurs, pregnant women are advised not to drink alcohol.

During breastfeeding, alcohol can also pass into a mother's milk.

It is best to avoid alcohol at this time. Mothers who want to have a drink should express milk for the next feed before drinking alcohol, and even then restrict their consumption to one glass.

How much?

Alcohol can have adverse effects on the developing brain so new advice recommends that teenagers do not drink. Government guidelines to help healthy men and women people stay below risky drinking levels state that:

- drinking no more than two standard drinks on any one day reduces the lifetime risk of harm from alcohol-related diseases or injury
- drinking no more than four standard drinks on any single occasion reduces the risk of alcohol-related diseases or injury arising from that occasion
- for pregnant women or those planning pregnancy and also those who are breastfeeding, not drinking is the safest option.

These guidelines do not apply to those with liver disease or anyone in charge of a car, bike, plane or boat, or operating machinery. People in these positions should avoid all alcohol. The guidelines also advise parents and carers of the importance of avoiding all alcohol for children under 15, and to delay starting drinking before 17 years for as long as possible.

Most health authorities advise people to have two alcohol-free days a week to guard against development of a dependence on alcohol.

Alcohol in cooking

Where wine or any other type of alcohol is used as an ingredient in cooking, some of the alcohol may be dissipated by heat. Nonetheless, some will remain, and the proportion depends on how long the dish is cooked. In general, if the alcohol is added at the end of cooking time, almost all of it is still present when the food is served. When brandy or rum or a liqueur is poured over a dish and set alight, about three-quarters of the alcohol remains. If you are serving a flaming dessert that will also be eaten by children, you can retain the effect by putting the alcohol in half an empty egg shell pushed into the dish. When sherry is added to a cold dessert such as trifle, almost three-quarters of the alcohol will be retained. Orange or raspberry juice make a suitable substitute for children. When alcohol is added to a casserole, about three-quarters will be lost after an hour of cooking; after two hours, very little will remain.

WHICH DRINK?

A standard drink contains 10 grams of alcohol. Some typical drinks pack a surprising punch.

Drink	Standard drink
Beer, regular, 375 mL (1 can)	1.5
Beer, light, 2.7% alcohol, 375 mL	0.8
Beer, regular, middy or pot, 285 mL	1
Light beer, 2.7% alcohol, middy or pot	0.5
Wine, red or white, average glass, 175 mL	2
Champagne, 160 mL	1.5
Port, 60 mL	1
Liqueur (e.g. Bailey's), 70 mL	1
Pre-mixed spirits (e.g. rum and cola), 375 mL can	1.5
Brandy, whisky, gin, 30 mL	1
Brandy, whisky, gin, 700 mL bottle	22

240

Yoghurt
– and probiotics

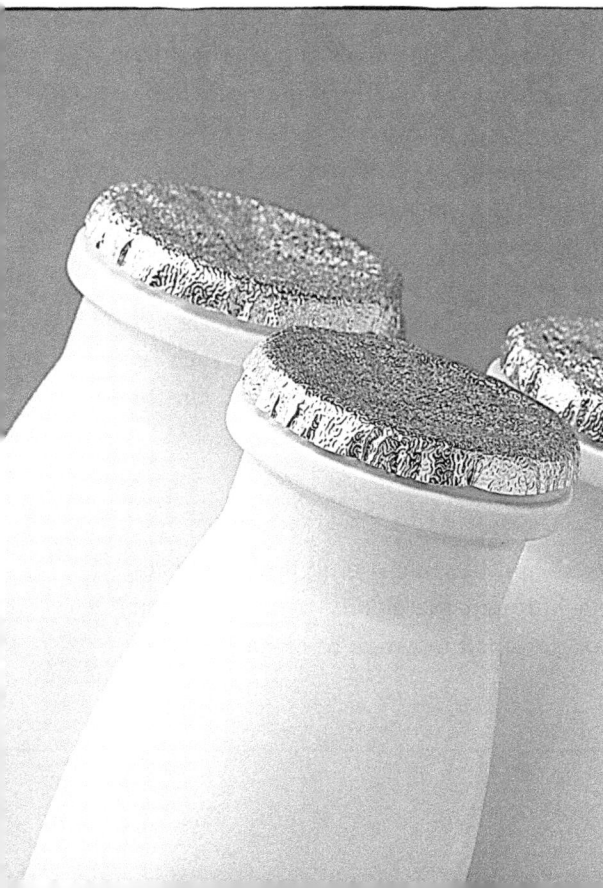

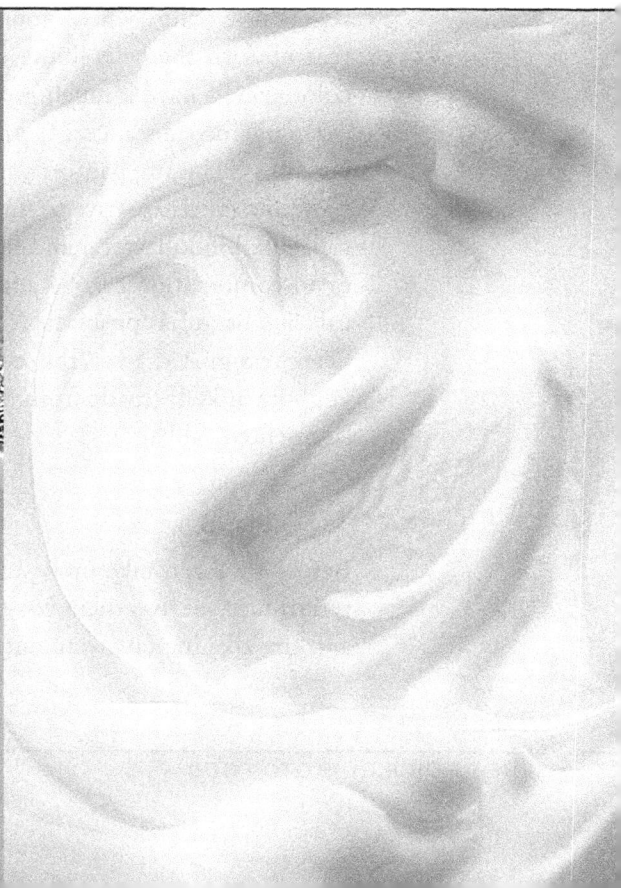

IT IS NOT SO LONG AGO that many Australians considered yoghurt a 'health food' purchased only by those of a slightly hippy bent. These days yoghurt is a mainstream product and highly regarded as a source of protein, calcium, riboflavin (vitamin B2), vitamin B12 and a range of other nutritional goodies. As yoghurt has become more popular, some varieties have acquired a hefty helping of added sugar, emulsifiers, thickeners and other additives. Others deserve the health status attributed to them, especially those that provide valuable live bacteria.

Probiotics

More than 100 years ago, scientists recognised that the protection against gastroenteritis enjoyed by breast-fed babies came from the bifidobacteria that dominated their gut microflora. More recently, microbiologists have identified over 500 species of beneficial bacteria in a healthy adult, with total numbers of these 'good bugs' hitting a mind-blowing 100 trillion. The helpful bacteria play many roles. Within the large intestine (colon), they break down dietary fibre from legumes, vegetables, fruits, whole grains, nuts and seeds, producing fatty acids that nourish the cells lining the intestine. The acids and the healthy colonic cells have a much greater chance of overthrowing potentially carcinogenic substances. Good bacteria in the intestine also synthesise vitamins K, biotin, pantothenic acid and even some vitamin B12.

Many scientists strive to find or develop particular strains of live lactobacilli, bifidobacteria and other beneficial bacteria that either singly or in combination can be added to foods for specific purposes. They call live bacteria 'probiotics'. The value of these healthy bacteria has been recognised over the centuries in traditional products such as yoghurt or kefir (made from milk), tempeh (fermented soy) and kimchi (fermented cabbage).

Prebiotics

Before they can take up residence and be truly useful, probiotic bacteria must survive their passage through the acidity of the stomach and the alkaline environment of the small intestine to reach the large intestine. Some substances can create an atmosphere that makes this environment more hospitable for probiotics, and these substances are now known as 'prebiotics'. Examples of prebiotics include the indigestible polysaccharides found in legumes, fruits such as bananas, some grains, and vegetables such as Jerusalem artichokes, onions, chicory and asparagus. One of these polysaccharides, inulin, can be extracted from artichokes or chicory root. Eager to produce foods that can make a claim to be healthier because they include prebiotics, manufacturers are now adding inulin and additives made from it to a wide range of foods, including yoghurt, cereals, drinks, low-fat desserts (where they also provide 'body') and foods and formula milks for infants. It is worth noting that a food with little or no nutritional value does not become healthy just because a prebiotic has been added.

Some yoghurts that do not contain fruit, such as vanilla flavoured or natural varieties, list some dietary fibre on their nutrition information panel. This comes from added inulin or one of its derivatives. Check the ingredient list. Inulin is also responsible for the various jokes that relate to production of gases after eating artichokes. The quantities of inulin added to many foods may be enough to cause wind.

The CSIRO has developed a strain of corn with a higher level of resistant starch that functions as a prebiotic. It is now added to breads, biscuits, cereals and snack foods. Pre- and probiotics are also sold as pills or powders, although there are no required tests for their usefulness.

Are there enough probiotics and prebiotics?

It's not easy to research pro- and prebiotics and progress has been much slower than some marketers would have us believe. Once you find beneficial bacteria that can actually get to the large intestine, the task is to sustain a bacterial colony that differs from the individual's normal microflora and is large enough to have a clinical effect. The Australian Food Standards Code stipulates that probiotic products must contain at least 1 million live bacteria per gram, but there is no universally recognised method of estimating live bacteria. Some tests by consumer groups have found that many yoghurts and fermented milk products do not have enough live bacteria to justify their probiotic claims.

Research into probiotics initially aimed to overcome the bugs that cause diarrhoea, a major problem for the world's poorest populations. The field has now widened with possibilities that probiotics may also help the body cope with inflammatory and immune responses. Researchers are studying the effects of specific probiotics on oral health, irritable bowel syndrome, inflammatory bowel disease, urinary tract infections, allergies and eczema.

At this stage, claims that probiotics will boost the immune system, bring inner harmony and treat food allergies and acne are premature. However, the combination of probiotics with rehydration fluids is showing some promise in treating rotavirus diarrhoea in children. The strains involved include *Lactobacillus GG, Lactobacillus casei, Bifidobacterium* spp., *Streptococcus* spp. and a yeast known as *Saccharomyces boulardii*. Some of these are now added to some brands of yoghurt. For traveller's diarrhoea, results have been mixed and limited. There is no evidence that probiotics have any effect on diarrhoea caused by bacteria rather than rotaviruses.

When do probiotics work?

ALLERGIES

Using probiotics to treat allergies is popular, but studies don't find long-term benefits when the probiotic is compared with placebo. One Finnish study that gave 1200 mothers from allergy-prone families either a probiotic mixture or a placebo during their pregnancy reported some possible benefits when the children were two but this had disappeared by five years of age. A major review has found no evidence supporting the use of probiotics for eczema.

IRRITABLE BOWEL SYNDROME

Many people who struggle to find an effective dietary treatment for irritable bowel syndrome have turned to probiotics – with some success. A particular strain of bifidobacteria appears to give some relief with improvements in gas, pain, bloating and diarrhoea.

INFLAMMATORY BOWEL DISEASE

At this stage, most studies using probiotics for Crohn's disease have found little benefit. Research using different strains of various bacteria is continuing. Results are more positive for a variety of probiotics, often combined with prebiotics, for treating ulcerative colitis and maintaining remission.

URINARY TRACT INFECTIONS

In theory, probiotics could inhibit bacteria in the urinary tract. Some early results look positive, and research is continuing.

DENTAL DECAY

Milk and products made from it, including yoghurt, contain natural compounds that help protect teeth from decay. Studies comparing probiotic dairy products containing lactobacilli and bifidobacteria with placebo products have found a reduction in the bacteria (*Mutans streptococci*) responsible for dental decay. Since filling the holes in children's teeth is the most expensive diet-related health problem in Australia (even greater than the costs associated with coronary heart disease), anything that reduces decay is of great benefit.

OTHER CONDITIONS

A major report from the Food and Agriculture Organization and the World Health Organization found no evidence that probiotics will improve the immune system. The authors also noted that claims probiotics (in yoghurt or other foods) will promote clearer skin, greater vitality, relief from common menopausal symptoms or a 'clean colon' are largely marketing hype.

Types of yoghurt

Check the ingredient list on yoghurt and choose those that contain milk and specified bacteria and as few other additives as possible. Avoid those with added sugar, thickeners, emulsifiers and numbered additives as their useful ingredients will have been diluted.

Natural yoghurt (sometimes called 'plain yoghurt') has 0–10 g fat/ 100 g and should have no added sugar. Check the ingredient list to

245

make sure. Natural yoghurt usually contains 5–6 g total sugar/100 g, with the slightly higher level appearing in low-fat products since most are made with concentrated skim milk to give them more 'body'.

Flavoured yoghurt varies according to the brand. Check the ingredient list. Vanilla yoghurt may have more added sugar than other flavours. The nutrition information panel will bundle the natural sugar in the yoghurt with any added sugar. Total sugars in vanilla yoghurts range from 10 g/100 g in full-fat to 12.5 g/100 g in low-fat products, indicating these products have 5–7 g of added sugar/100 g. Fruit flavoured yoghurts have a content of total sugars of about 11 g/100 g for full-fat with low-fat flavoured varieties having about 13 g/100 g. The extra 8 g of sugar on top of the natural milk sugar comes from added sugar as well as any fruit content. Fruit yoghurts must tell you the percentage of the fruit named on the label, but this may be obscured if the fruit comes from fruit puree or fruit juice concentrate, which has few of the nutrients from the original fruit. Adding your own fruit to natural yoghurt gives a more nutritious mixture.

Greek-style yoghurt is regular yoghurt that has been drained so that it is thicker and thus higher in all nutrients and kilojoules per 100 g. Some varieties also include cream to add to the texture. As with other products, check the ingredient list.

The take-home message

It makes good nutritional sense to include highly nutritious foods such as yoghurt or other fermented dairy products in the diet and continuing research is likely to identify more specific bacterial strains with particular uses. However, there is insufficient evidence to back many of the claims made by the sellers of some probiotic products.

The following resources are useful. The books should be available in most libraries. Note that diet books, and misinformation on the internet, abound.

Internet sites

GENERAL NUTRITION

CHOICE **www.choice.com.au**
Food Politics **www.foodpolitics.com**
Nutrition Australia **www.nutritionaustralia.org**
Public Health Victoria **www.health.vic.gov.au**
Queensland Health **www.health.qld.gov.au**
Health *Insite* **www.healthinsite.gov.au**
Centre for Health Promotion South Australia
    www.healthpromotion.cywhs.sa.gov.au
Dietitians Association of Australia **www.daa.asn.au**
Quackwatch **www.quackwatch.com**

NUTRITION AND CHILDREN

Cancer Council Junk Food Injunction
    www.cancercouncil.com.au/cfac/junkfoodinjunction.html
The Coalition on Food Advertising to Children **www.cfac.net.au**
The Parents Jury **www.parentsjury.org.au**

OBESITY

The Obesity Coalition **www.opc.org.au**

FOOD AND THE ENVIRONMENT

The Climate Institute **www.climateinstitute.org.au**
Marine Stewardship Council **www.msc.org**
Institute of Sustainable Futures, University of Technology Sydney
    www.isf.uts.edu.au
Food Fairness Alliance **www.sydneyfoodfairness.org.au**

BOOKS AND MAGAZINES

CHOICE Magazine, Australia
Cribb, Julian, *The coming famine*, CSIRO Publishing, Melbourne, 2010.
Farrell, David, *Great wealth, poor health*, Copyright Publishing, Brisbane, 2009.
Gabriel, Yiannis & Lang, Tim, *The unmanageable consumer*, Sage Publications, London, 1995.

Gussow, Joan Dye, *This organic life: confessions of a suburban homesteader*, Chelsea Green Publishing, White River Junction, VT, 2001.

Kausman, Rick, *If not dieting, then what?* Allen & Unwin, Sydney, 1998.

Nestle, Marion, *Food politics*, University of California Press, Berkeley, 2002.

Pollan, Michael, *The omnivore's dilemma*, Penguin Press, New York, 2006.

Pollan, Michael, *In defence of food*, Allen Lane, Melbourne, 2008.

Roberts, Paul, *The end of food*, Bloomsbury, London, 2009.

Schlosser, Eric, *Fast food nation*, Allen Lane, London, 2001.

Skurray, Geoffrey, *Decoding food additives*, Lothian Books, Sydney, 2006.

Stanton, Rosemary, *Rosemary Stanton's complete book of food and nutrition*, Simon & Schuster, Sydney, 2007.